Telehealth in Sleep Medicine

Editors

DENNIS HWANG
JEAN-LOUIS PÉPIN

SLEEP MEDICINE CLINICS

www.sleep.theclinics.com

Consulting Editor
TEOFILO LEE-CHIONG Jr

September 2020 • Volume 15 • Number 3

ELSEVIER

1600 John F. Kennedy Boulevard • Suite 1800 • Philadelphia, Pennsylvania, 19103-2899

http://www.theclinics.com

SLEEP MEDICINE CLINICS Volume 15, Number 3
September 2020, ISSN 1556-407X, ISBN-13: 978-0-323-72224-7

Editor: John Vassallo
Developmental Editor: Donald Mumford

Sleep Medicine Clinics (ISSN 1556-407X) is published quarterly by Elsevier Inc., 360 Park Avenue South, New York, NY 10010-1710. Months of issue are March, June, September and December. Business and Editorial Offices: 1600 John F. Kennedy Blvd., Ste. 1800, Philadelphia, PA 19103-2899. Customer Service Office: 3251 Riverport Lane, Maryland Heights, MO 63043. Periodicals postage paid at New York, NY and additional mailing offices. Subscription prices are $218.00 per year (US individuals), $100.00 (US and Canadian students), $518.00 (US institutions), $264.00 (Canadian individuals), $252.00 (international individuals), $135.00 (International students), $587.00 (Canadian and International institutions). Foreign air speed delivery is included in all *Clinics* subscription prices. All prices are subject to change without notice. **POSTMASTER:** Send change of address to *Sleep Medicine Clinics*, Elsevier Health Sciences Division, Subscription Customer Service, 3251 Riverport Lane, Maryland Heights, MO 63043. Customer Service: **Tel: 1-800-654-2452 (U.S. and Canada); 314-447-8871 (outside U.S. and Canada). Fax: 314-447-8029. E-mail: journalscustomerservice-usa@elsevier.com (for print support); journalsonline-support-usa@elsevier.com (for online support)**.

Reprints. For copies of 100 or more of articles in this publication, please contact the Commercial Reprints Department, Elsevier Inc., 360 Park Avenue South, New York, NY 10010-1710. Tel.: 212-633-3874; Fax: 212-633-3820; E-mail: reprints@elsevier.com.

Sleep Medicine Clinics is covered in *MEDLINE/PubMed (Index Medicus)*.

SLEEP MEDICINE CLINICS

SERIES OF RELATED INTEREST

Clinics in Chest Medicine
Available at: https://www.chestmed.theclinics.com/

THE CLINICS ARE AVAILABLE ONLINE!
Access your subscription at:
www.theclinics.com

SLEEP MEDICINE CLINICS

Contributors

CONSULTING EDITOR

TEOFILO LEE-CHIONG, Jr, MD
Professor of Medicine, National Jewish Health;
Professor of Medicine, University of Colorado,
Denver, Colorado, USA; Chief Medical Liaison,
Philips Respironics, Pennsylvania, USA

EDITORS

DENNIS HWANG, MD
Medical Director, Kaiser Permanente SBC
Sleep Medicine, Internal Medicine, Pulmonary,
and Critical Care; Co-Chair, Sleep Medicine,
Southern California Medical Group, Fontana,
California, USA

JEAN-LOUIS PÉPIN, MD, PhD
Grenoble Alpes University Hospital, HP2,
Inserm U1042, Grenoble, France

AUTHORS

FARIHA ABBASI-FEINBERG, MD, FAASM
Medical Director of Sleep Medicine, Millennium
Physician Group, Fort Myers, Florida, USA

TEREZA CERVENKA, MD
Assistant Professor, Department of Medicine,
Division of Pulmonary, Allergy, Critical Care
and Sleep Medicine, M Health Fairview and
University of Minnesota, Minneapolis,
Minnesota, USA

WALTER D. CONWELL, MD, MBA
Associate Dean for Equity, Inclusion, and
Diversity, Assistant Professor, Department of
Clinical Science, Kaiser Permanente Bernard J.
Tyson School of Medicine, Pasadena,
California, USA

BARRY G. FIELDS, MD, MSEd
Associate Professor of Medicine, Department
of Pulmonary, Allergy, Critical Care, and Sleep
Medicine, Emory University School of
Medicine, Atlanta VA Health Care System,
Atlanta, Georgia, USA

CATHY GOLDSTEIN, MD, MS
Associate Professor of Neurology, University of
Michigan Sleep Disorders Center, Ann Arbor,
Michigan, USA

CALEB HSIEH, MD, MS
Pulmonary, Critical Care and Sleep Medicine,
David Geffen School of Medicine at UCLA, Los
Angeles, California, USA

CONRAD IBER, MD
Professor of Medicine and Sleep Medicine
Section Director, Department of Medicine,
Division of Pulmonary, Allergy, Critical Care
and Sleep Medicine, M Health Fairview and
University of Minnesota, Minneapolis,
Minnesota, USA

NIKKY KEER, DO
Sleep Medicine Fellow, Division of Pulmonary,
Critical Care, and Sleep Medicine, Department
of Medicine, The University of Tennessee
Health Science Center, College of Medicine,
Memphis, Tennessee, USA

SEEMA KHOSLA, MD, FCCP, FAASM
Medical Director, ND Center for Sleep,
Fargo, North Dakota, USA

WALTER T. McNICHOLAS, MD, FERS
Department of Respiratory and Sleep
Medicine, School of Medicine, University
College Dublin, St. Vincent's University
Hospital, St. Vincent's Hospital Group, Dublin,
Ireland

BURTON N. MELIUS, MBA
Senior Manager, Consulting and
Implementation, Southern California
Permanente Medical Group, Pasadena,
California, USA

CLIONA O'DONNELL, MB BCh BAO
UCD School of Medicine, Health Sciences
Centre, University College Dublin, Belfield,
Dublin, Ireland; Department of Respiratory and
Sleep Medicine, St. Vincent's University
Hospital, Elm Park, Dublin, Ireland

TALAYEH REZAYAT, DO, MPH
Pulmonary, Critical Care and Sleep Medicine,
David Geffen School of Medicine at UCLA Los
Angeles, California, USA

SILKE RYAN, MD, PhD
UCD School of Medicine, Health Sciences
Centre, University College Dublin, Belfield,
Dublin, Ireland; Department of Respiratory and
Sleep Medicine, St. Vincent's University
Hospital, Elm Park, Dublin, Ireland

**SHARON SCHUTTE-RODIN, MD, DABSM,
FAASM, CBSM**
Adjunct Professor of Medicine, University of
Pennsylvania Perelman School of Medicine,
Penn Sleep Center, Philadelphia,
Pennsylvania, USA

JASPAL SINGH, MD, MHA, MHS, FAASM
Professor of Medicine, Atrium Health and
Levine Cancer Institute, Carolinas Medical
Center and Atrium Health, Charlotte, North
Carolina, USA

MICHELLE R. ZEIDLER, MD, MS
Pulmonary, Critical Care and Sleep Medicine,
David Geffen School of Medicine at UCLA, Los
Angeles, California, USA

Contents

Telemedicine is about more than simply using audio-visual technology to care for patients, but rather an opportunity to fundamentally improve patient access, quality, efficiencies, and experience. Regarding sleep medicine, it has the potential to drive sleep medicine's evolution. By enabling care across geographies and facilitating population-based management, sleep medicine is poised to take advantage of telemedicine capabilities. In this introductory chapter, we highlight issues related to sleep telemedicine, while providing a framework in which to approach this transformational journey thoughtfully. We thereby set the stage for the individual chapters in this edition of Sleep Medicine Clinics.

Synchronous telemedicine allows clinicians to expand their reach by using technology to take care of patients who otherwise may not be seen. Establishing a telemedicine practice can be daunting. This article outlines how to implement a synchronous telemedicine practice into an existing workflow. Telemedicine-specific considerations are discussed, as well as guidance regarding practice assessment, financial feasibility, technical considerations, and clinical guidance to translate in-person visit skills into an effective virtual visit.

Obstructive sleep apnea (OSA) telehealth management may improve initial and chronic care access, time to diagnosis and treatment, between-visit care, e-communications and e-education, workflows, costs, and therapy outcomes. OSA telehealth options may be used to replace or supplement none, some, or all steps in the evaluation, testing, treatments, and management of OSA. All telehealth steps must adhere to OSA guidelines. OSA telehealth may be adapted for continuous positive airway pressure (CPAP) and non-CPAP treatments. E-data collection enhances uses for individual and group analytics, phenotyping, testing and treatment selections, high-risk identification and targeted support, and comparative and multispecialty therapy studies.

EHR optimization facilitates continuous care population telehealth care in sleep medicine. Positive airway pressure (PAP) therapy integration can facilitate continuity and efficiency as a component of this optimization accross health care systems. In an operating clinical model with EHR device integration and sleep medicine optimization, a patient-centered coordinated care plan can also leverage monitoring and timely telehealth interventions.

The Impact of Telehealth on the Organization of the Health System and Integrated Care   431

Cliona O'Donnell, Silke Ryan, and Walter T. McNicholas

Sleep medicine is a rapidly developing field of medicine that is well-suited to initiatives such as Telehealth to provide safe, effective clinical care to an expanding group of patients. The increasing prevalence of sleep disorders has resulted in long waiting lists and lack of specialist availability. Telemedicine has potential to facilitate a move toward an integrated care model, which involves professionals from different disciplines and different organizations working together in a team-oriented way toward a shared goal of delivering all of a person's care requirements. Issues around consumer health technology and nonphysician sleep providers are discussed further in the article.

Impact of Telehealth on Health Economics   441

Burton N. Melius and Walter D. Conwell

As part of an efficient, continuously improving care delivery system, telehealth can increase patient engagement by creating new or additional ways of communicating with patients' physicians. Telehealth has the potential to increase patient and primary care provider access to specialists, provide specialist support to rural providers, assist with on-going monitoring and support for patients with chronic conditions, and reduce health care expenses by maximizing the use of specialists without the need to duplicate coverage in multiple locations. Current and future physicians will need to develop competencies that will enable them to navigate this new telehealth landscape.

Sleep medicine is a rapidly developing field of medicine that is well suited to initiatives such as Telehealth to provide safe, effective clinical care to an expanding group of patients. The increasing prevalence of sleep disorders has resulted in long waiting lists and lack of specialist availability. Telemedicine has potential to facilitate a move toward an integrated care model, which involves professionals from different disciplines and different organizations working together in a team-oriented way toward a shared goal of delivering all of a person's care requirements. Issues around consumer health technology and nonphysician sleep providers are discussed further in the article.

As part of an efficient, continuously improving care delivery system, telehealth can increase patient engagement by creating new or additional ways of communicating with patients, physicians. Telehealth has the potential to increase patient and primary care provider access to specialists, provide specialist support to rural providers, assist with on-going monitoring and support for patients with chronic conditions, and reduce health care expenses by maximizing the use of specialists without the need to duplicate coverage in multiple locations. Current and future physicians will need to develop competencies that will enable them to navigate this new telehealth landscape.

Preface

Sleep Telemedicine: A Template for Other Specialties?

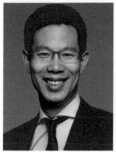 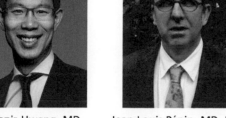

Dennis Hwang, MD   Jean-Louis Pépin, MD, PhD

Editors

On March 18, 2020, the doors to our sleep center were physically closed. As with so many other sleep centers worldwide in response to COVID-19, our service transitioned completely to virtual care while care providers were moved to "work from home." It was perhaps that moment that we felt the emotional impact that the world had changed, altering both our personal lives and sleep medicine as we knew it. This event also presented a transformative opportunity to reimagine our identity, accelerating the efforts to bring the future of sleep medicine into the present. Innovation progress in health care tends to be deliberate, proceeding at an incremental pace built upon business cases, challenges related to funding and financial incentives, and health care infrastructure barriers. Many of those hurdles dissolved once COVID-19 intensified, exemplified by rapid approval of video visit encounter reimbursements in the United States and intense support toward implementing remote patient monitoring technologies.

In this issue of *Sleep Medicine Clinics*, thought leaders in our field provide their vision for the application of innovative synchronous and nonsynchronous technology-based tools. Practical discussions to help navigate implementation of telehealth (eg, video visits) in various populations are provided along with creative discussions projecting the development and application of remote patient monitoring and artificial intelligence. The current health care environment embodies the principle to "never let a serious crisis go to waste." During this pandemic, we have been afforded a taste of the future of sleep medicine. Strategies such as population management, intelligent personalized care, longitudinal remote monitoring with wearable devices, and machine learning–derived clinical decision tools have transitioned from abstract ideas into practical tools actively impacting patient care. This period may be the inflection point for an evolutionary shift in sleep medicine based upon the experience and insights gained from this transition. If our field can successfully navigate implementation and validate the impact of these telehealth strategies, sleep medicine could represent a template for other specialties in innovating chronic care disease management. We hope that the expertise presented in this issue will be an important resource in facilitating this journey.

Dennis Hwang, MD
Fontana Medical Center
9961 Sierra Avenue, MOB7
Fontana, CA 92335, USA

Jean-Louis Pépin, MD, PhD
Laboratoire EFCR/Pneumologie
CHU Grenoble Alpes, Site Nord
Hôpital Couple Enfant
Boulevard de la Chantourne CS10217
Grenoble Cedex 9 38043, France

E-mail addresses:
Dennis.X.Hwang@kp.org (D. Hwang)
JPepin@chu-grenoble.fr (J.-L. Pépin)

Sleep Med Clin 15 (2020) xi
https://doi.org/10.1016/j.jsmc.2020.07.001
1556-407X/20/© 2020 Published by Elsevier Inc.

Overview of Telemedicine and Sleep Disorders

Jaspal Singh, MD, MHA, MHS[a],*, Nikky Keer, DO[b]

KEYWORDS

- Telemedicine • Telehealth • Virtual care • Sleep • Download • Data integration

KEY POINTS

- There is a clear need for the sleep medicine provider to consider telehealth use, and find means for incorporating, integrating, and expanding telehealth strategies.
- The technology behind telemedicine integration is often less of a consideration than strategic design of the telemedicine practice (workflow design, logistics, and communication).
- The telehealth industry's rapid and expansive growth, coupled with evolving legislation and reimbursement schemes, requires attention and consideration when defining the technology and applications.
- Individual articles provide a more comprehensive examination of the various aspects of sleep telehealth adoption and integration.
- Important questions related to telehealth still need to be answered, including what is the true impact of telehealth on quality, access, and efficiencies of sleep medicine? What is the impact of telehealth on individual patient and provider experiences?

INTRODUCTION

We are delighted to introduce this edition of *Sleep Medicine Clinics*, which focuses on telemedicine and its applications, whereby multiple authors provide important and unique insights to the issues surrounding sleep telehealth as this field evolves. In this introduction, we provide a clinical, organizational, and philosophic context to the incorporation of sleep telehealth. To us and many others, telemedicine for sleep disorders is a natural fit, because:

- There is a large unmet patient need for sleep specialists that may be partially allayed by the expansion of telemedicine.
- Diagnostic and treatment algorithms of several common disorders like obstructive sleep apnea are often data driven, enabling sound clinical decision making, potentially even in the absence of a physical examination.
- Sleep clinicians generally rely less on discrete physical examination findings than many other specialists.
- Telemedicine may minimize some of the traditional barriers that have hindered the growth of sleep medicine as a specialty.

Given these and other issues related to rapid technological adoption by society in general, sleep medicine seems poised to build on this platform of patient care delivery.

CONTENT

The telemedicine industry is growing, and even before the coronavirus disease-2019 (COVID-19)

[a] Atrium Health and Levine Cancer Institute, Carolinas Medical Center and Atrium Health, 1000 Blythe Boulevard, 506B Medical Education Building, Charlotte, NC 28203, USA; [b] Division of Pulmonary, Critical Care, and Sleep Medicine, Department of Medicine, University of Tennessee HSC COM at Memphis, Suite H316B, 956 Court Avenue, Memphis, TN 38163, USA
* Corresponding author.
E-mail address: Jaspal.Singh@atriumhealth.org
Twitter: @Singh011Jaspal (J.S.); @nikkykeer (N.K.)

Sleep Med Clin 15 (2020) 341–346
https://doi.org/10.1016/j.jsmc.2020.05.005
1556-407X/20/© 2020 Elsevier Inc. All rights reserved.

pandemic, the market was expected to hit $53.1 billion by 2026 in a recent report from Acumen Research and Consulting.[1] Fueled by faster data streaming options, better camera resolution, and enhanced software features, the technical aspects seem positioned optimally for telemedicine to succeed. In fact, since COVID-19 and the widespread adoption of telemedicine to provide care while practicing social distancing, we expect those figures to skyrocket.[2] The frenetic pace at which primary care and specialties adopt telemedicine practices has been nothing short of breathtaking for telemedicine enthusiasts. It is also quite possible that the COVID-19 pandemic and the Medicare CARES Act have changed the face of telemedicine for the foreseeable future.

So, if adequate technology is ubiquitous, why has telemedicine for sleep practices been so slow to evolve? It has been slowed down not only by previous issues of low reimbursement and slow adoption of technology, but also several key issues related to workflow disruption, behavioral and psychological issues, and of course disparities in access to technology.[3] As such, the array of services, user functionalities, and payment and workflow schemes have left many confused, and perhaps overwhelmed, by where to begin. There are many unique factors to health care regulation, many players and stakeholders, and a host of issues related to change management difficulties. Thus, it has been difficult to identify clear

paths to success as the pace of the technology, consumer demand, and regulatory and financial issues are continually evolving. Such rapid and constant change are almost akin to playing a high-stakes game while one is actively learning the rules; moreover, the rules keep changing. With all these factors, it is no wonder many sleep medicine clinicians have been less keen to adopt and incorporate telehealth.

Sleep medicine has been exposed previously to large-scale disruption, because home sleep apnea testing was met by years of intense resistance.[4,5] This change finally led to broader acceptance and integration into the daily practice of a sleep practitioner, benefitting a countless number of patients. Many would suggest sleep medicine as a field benefitted from incorporation of new technology. In this vein, we would in fact argue that it is once again in the best interest of the field to accept this tidal wave of change by broad adoption and incorporation of telehealth into the sleep provider's clinical operations. We believe this has the potential to clearly benefit patients, sleep practices, and create much larger and broader impact through several potential mechanisms as discussed in this issue of *Sleep Medicine Clinics* (**Fig. 1**). However, the logistics of telemedicine, including its nuances, need to be understood. Importantly, one must also consider a patient-centered approach while maintaining fiscal, ethical, and legal responsibilities.

Benefits of Sleep Telehealth from *Patient* Perspective	Benefits of Sleep Telehealth from *Provider's* Perspective	Benefits of Sleep Telehealth from *Population or Healthcare System* Perspective
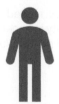	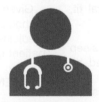	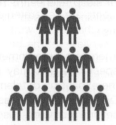
• Convenient visits • Fewer barriers to care • Use existing tools to monitor • Personalize care through technology • Timely feedback and interaction	• Minimize distance travel • Customize apps to practice needs • Potential to manage larger panel • Increased abilities to supervise APPs, incorporate team members • Unique opportunities for coding, billing, practice growth	• Provide effective team-based communication and coordination • Integrate care with EHR, data analytics • Incorporate decision-support systems and AI • Drive large-scale initiative and complex care mechanisms

Fig. 1. The potential benefits of sleep telehealth from different perspectives. The use of telehealth has the ability to benefit a number of different key participants in unique ways. AI, artificial intelligence; APP, advanced practice provider (eg, nurse practitioner, physician assistant); EHR, electronic health record.

As background, in 2015, the American Academy of Sleep Medicine published its Position Paper for the Use of Telemedicine for the Diagnosis and Treatment of Sleep Disorders,[6] to seek more efficient and accessible ways to provide services beyond the traditional office model. The Position Paper noted that, at time of publication, the expansion of sleep telemedicine into all aspects of sleep disorder management was limited by technology resources and reimbursement and financial considerations, as well as a willingness of physicians, patients, and health care organizations to accept telemedicine as an alternative to in-office care.[6] In this edition of *Sleep Medicine Clinics*, the editors have assembled a thoughtful group of experts who have a great deal of pragmatic experience in each of their areas, so that readers can learn other success factors (and some difficult lessons) in sleep telehealth use.

Defining Sleep Telehealth

Because telemedicine is often referred to mean different models of care delivery, a quick recap of the definitions might be worth noting. The American Telemedicine Association cites 4 key models of telemedicine services: synchronous and asynchronous (store-and-forward) telemedicine patient encounters, remote patient monitoring (RPM), and mobile health (mHealth) smartphone applications. Each of these receives a thorough examination in this edition, with pragmatic advice provided by each of the authors. For some basic definitions:

- *Synchronous telemedicine* refers to the delivery of a live, interactive encounter in which patients and providers are separated by distance but interact in real-time using video-conferencing as the core technology. Participants are separated by distance but interact synchronously with the provider performing interviews of the patient, and diagnostic and treatment options are addressed through live video interaction between the patient and the provider.
- *Asynchronous (store-and-forward) telemedicine* is defined as a non–real-time, technology-assisted exchange of structured information between a patient and provider with the intent to diagnose, treat, and/or triage. For example, a sleep medicine history with certain diagnostic/therapeutic data are collected at the point of care and transmitted to the sleep medicine provider for review. In turn, the sleep medicine specialist provides clinical advice via a written or electronic report to the referring provider within a reasonable time frame to make clinical decisions.

- *RPM* refers to the use of digital devices to remotely collect physiologic data for interpretation and management of a patient under a specific treatment plan. For example, telemonitoring is routinely performed of positive airway pressure use; however, increasing RPM of physical activity, oximetry, or ambulatory blood pressure by the sleep clinician may also be considered. As such, this situation has to the potential to lead to personalized care, more rapid and frequent assessments, and perhaps even behavioral change. In addition, this technology may be used to do drive complex disease management to care for high-risk patients with a mix of cardiopulmonary and neuropsychiatric disorders. Such applications have been shown to be successful in a broad range of disease states.
- *Mobile health applications, or mHealth,* encompasses personal computer and smartphone applications that may be used to provide individuals with the behavioral and cognitive skills to manage a disease process. The application of sensors, mobile apps, and location tracking technology may not only enable simple behavioral changes, but also allow monitoring and intervention whenever and wherever acute and chronic medical conditions occur.

Arguably, RPM and mHealth models represent a heterogenous spectrum between asynchronous telemedicine and self-directed care mechanisms. However, these are worth mentioning now.

Importantly, the use of telehealth provides the opportunity therefore for responsive feedback from the patient and/or population, while setting the stage for more complex disease and population management schemes. It also creates interesting dilemmas as the lines become increasingly blurred between defining when a patient encounter begins and ends, which is why it is imperative to understand the technical, legal, regulatory, and financial environments in which one develops telehealth strategies.

The Workforce Issue

Incorporation of sleep telehealth has the inherent potential to allow the limited number of specialists in the workforce to serve the broader population. The Centers for Disease Control and Prevention estimate that 50 to 70 million of the general adult population in the United States suffers from chronic disease related to sleep deficiency and sleep disorders. The repercussions of sleep deficiency include disease burden, lost productivity and accidents, and an array of social determinants underlying health and health disparities. Fortunately, the general public is more aware than ever before of the importance of healthy sleep. Employers are placing a greater value on sleep and insurers, regulators, and legislators recognize the importance of diagnosing and treating sleep disorders. However, as of 2018, there are 6035 sleep medicine physicians board certified by the American Board of Medical Specialties.[7] The reality is that this workforce is insufficient to meet the demands of the enormous population of patients who have a sleep disorder. By leveraging telemedicine capabilities, sleep physicians can access patients that who be in more rural or remote locations and increase access to subspecialties within sleep (eg, pediatric sleep experts, dental sleep experts), while allowing those practitioners to save time and costs associated with travel or distant clinics.

Importantly, telemedicine truly allows sleep providers to serve more as team leaders in the care of patients, allowing for potentially a greater population served. Studies conducted within closed health care systems such as the Veterans Administration system[8] or Kaiser Permanente[9] have provided data on the value of telehealth components for evaluation and treatment, and how these components are delivered. Telehealth use has led to dramatically reduced wait-times from referral to diagnosis and treatment of sleep-related breathing disorders as well as increased adherence to treatment, despite an increase in the volume of sleep consults and sleep studies performed.[8,9]

Questions remain, however, about whether the workforce can adapt to these pressures. Will telemedicine allow these providers to adopt, sustain, and grow larger panels of patients? Will such providers be skilled and enabled to lead care teams through virtual access tools? Will regulations and payment schemes limit successes in different markets of this approach? These are important questions that need to be addressed from the workforce perspective on the use of telemedicine.

Financial Considerations

Reimbursement has been and is one of the most significant barriers to the implementation of telehealth nationwide. Encouragingly, state and federal legislation and regulation have been increasingly broadening access to telehealth services in recent years. In 2019, 48 state Medicaid programs were reimbursing for synchronous video-based telehealth. Additionally, 40 states and the District of Columbia had adopted substantive policies to expand telehealth coverage and reimbursement. Furthermore, the Centers for Medicare and Medicaid Services has shown a

dedication to support these policies by continually expanding its fee schedule to reimburse newer forms of telehealth. For example, Current Procedural Terminology codes to support RPM of physiologic values were added to the 2019 Medicare Physician Fee Schedule. Even before the COVID-19 pandemic, there had been rapid adoption, acceptance, and even demand of telehealth by both physicians and patients. A study of more than 29 billion private health care claim records found that national use of telehealth grew tremendously between 2014 and 2018.[10] In particular, the number of non–hospital-based provider-to-patient telehealth claims increased at a rate of an astonishing 1393%, much greater than other types of telehealth claims (**Fig. 2**).

Investment opportunities in telehealth have also been rapidly expanding. Remarkably, digital health received nearly 1 in 10 venture dollars invested in the United States in 2019, totaling more than $7 billion.[11] Additionally, digital health companies are proving outcomes and cost validation, increasing the likelihood of success when these ventures enter the public market. As of January 1, 2020, the combined market cap of the 9 digital health companies that entered the public market in 2019 is a staggering $17 billion.[11] There are countless applications currently on the market to provide an array of telehealth solutions, and likely more to come soon. Importantly, in 2016 the American Academy of Sleep Medicine even launched its own sleep telemedicine platform, SleepTM. This platform provides services ranging from synchronous telemedicine encounters for sleep disordered breathing, cognitive behavioral therapy for insomnia as well as data management and coordination of care services for durable medical equipment. With the dizzying pace of technological innovation, the US Food and Drug Administration has enacted a Digital Health Innovation Action Plan to provide regulatory framework for medical device software, mHealth, and other platforms. The goal is to provide timely patient access to high-quality, safe, and effective medical technology.

Regardless of telehealth strategy and application(s), the financial implications for payers, industry, investors, and the consumers will be scrutinized closely. As much as telemedicine offers a lot to be gained, concerns of costs, integration, and usability still will remain. Moreover, the current reimbursement scheme by the Centers for Medicare and Medicaid Services is in response to the COVID-19 pandemic, which if the reimbursement changes afterward, or the health care sector economy collapses,[12] then telemedicine may not be as easy to sustain in the current

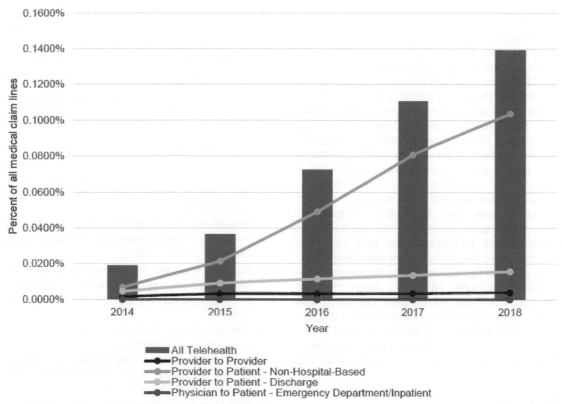

Fig. 2. Claim lines with telehealth usage by type as a percentage of all medical claim lines. (Source: "A Multilayered Analysis of Telehealth" [June 2019]. © FAIR Health, Inc. Reprinted with permission.)

projections. Much is evolving in this landscape as the financial sectors brace for a post–COVID-19 world, and sleep telemedicine is not immune to the market forces.

How to Navigate This Issue of Sleep Medicine Clinics

This issue of *Sleep Medicine Clinics* offers a complete review of key principles related to sleep telemedicine. After the introduction, this edition begins with implementation of synchronous telemedicine, a staple for most sleep telemedicine provider's approach. Therefore, understanding the practical aspects of the telemedicine or virtual visit is an imperative for the sleep professional. This is then followed by a thoughtful discussion of how one approaches the electronic health record, integration with data systems, and population management tools in sleep medicine. Subsequent articles expand on the introduction of consumer sleep technologies and device wearables mentioned elsewhere in this issue, providing the reader with insight into the rapid advancements that many sleep clinicians see daily in their offices. After this overview, further detail is provided regarding how to

manage certain populations with common sleep disorders such as obstructive sleep apnea and insomnia, with the respective authors providing tremendous insight and pragmatic information including managing those with complex interrelated disease states. This issue also addresses how to use telehealth to better integrate nonphysician providers, facilitate team-based care, and even what unique teaching and research opportunities are afforded using telemedicine. Importantly, in-depth evaluations of regulatory, legal, and ethics issues as well as important principles related to coding, reimbursement, and financial considerations are highlighted. Last, the integration of predictive analytics as the concluding article leads us into the many possibilities that telemedicine with all its uses and applications may allow.

We are excited about this edition, particularly as each author is not only an accomplished leader, but also a skilled clinician. As such, each author has tried (and failed) at certain aspects of telemedicine care delivery, but each wants the next person to be successful in advancing the field as well as the care of any patient with a sleep disorder.

SUMMARY

Telemedicine is growing rapidly in all aspects of medicine, and sleep medicine seems well-poised to adapt to this transformation of health care delivery. That said, there are numerous issues related to understanding the technologies, the interface, the workflow and the patient and provider experience. Last, providing value, and remaining fiscally, legally, and ethically responsible are important considerations with the sleep telemedicine. Therefore, in this issue of *Sleep Medicine Clinics*, a collection of articles has been assembled that address where our field currently is with respect to telemedicine and telehealth principles for many sleep disorders. It is our opinion that sleep telehealth will be synonymous and integrated with bedside care of the patient with sleep disorders, and that the time is now to incorporate telemedicine principles into one's sleep medicine practice. But there remain questions as to how and to what degree sleep telemedicine will affect the quality, access, and efficiencies of the care of the sleep patient, and to what lessons the sleep medicine field will learn and share along this journey.

DISCLOSURE

J. Singh is on the Physician Advisory Board of Somnoware Sleep Solutions, Inc.

REFERENCES

1. Smith R. Telehealth market to hit $53.1 billion by 2026. Insurance Business America Web site. 2020. Available at: https://www.insurancebusinessmag.com/us/news/breaking-news/telehealth-market-to-hit-53-1-billion-by-2026–report-213866.aspx. Accessed May 5, 2020.
2. Hollander JE, Carr BG. Virtually perfect? telemedicine for COVID-19. N Engl J Med 2020;382(18):1679–81.
3. Kane CK, Gillis K. The use of telemedicine by physicians: still the exception rather than the rule. Health Aff (Millwood) 2018;37(12):1923–30.
4. Tan HL, Kheirandish-Gozal L, Gozal D. Pediatric home sleep apnea testing: slowly getting there! Chest 2015;148(6):1382–95.
5. Collop NA. Portable monitoring for the diagnosis of obstructive sleep apnea. Curr Opin Pulm Med 2008;14(6):525–9.
6. Singh J, Badr MS, Diebert W, et al. American Academy of Sleep Medicine (AASM) position paper for the use of telemedicine for the diagnosis and treatment of sleep disorders. J Clin Sleep Med 2015;11(10):1187–98.
7. Kiley JP, Twery MJ, Gibbons GH. The national center on sleep disorders research-progress and promise. Sleep 2019;42(6):zsz105.
8. Sarmiento KF, Folmer RL, Stepnowsky CJ, et al. National expansion of sleep telemedicine for veterans: the telesleep program. J Clin Sleep Med 2019;15(9):1355–64.
9. Hwang D, Chang JW, Benjafield AV, et al. Effect of telemedicine education and telemonitoring on continuous positive airway pressure adherence. the tele-OSA randomized trial. Am J Respir Crit Care Med 2018;197(1):117–26.
10. FAIRHealth A. Multilayered Analysis of telehealth 2019. Available at: https://s3.amazonaws.com/media2.fairhealth.org/whitepaper/asset/A%20Multilayered%20Analysis%20of%20Telehealth%20-%20A%20FAIR%20Health%20White%20Paper.pdf. Accessed January 15, 2020.
11. Day S, Gambon E. In 2019, digital health celebrated six IPOs as venture investment edged off record highs. Rock Health. Available at: https://rockhealth.com/reports/in-2019-digital-health-celebrated-six-ipos-as-venture-investment-edged-off-record-highs/. Accessed January 15, 2020.
12. Barnett ML, Mehrotra A, Landon BE. Covid-19 and the upcoming financial crisis in health care. NEJM Catal 2020.

Implementation of Synchronous Telemedicine into Clinical Practice

Seema Khosla, MD, FCCP*

KEYWORDS

- Telemedicine • Telehealth • Synchronous • Center to home • Center to center • E-visit • Telemed
- Web-side manner

KEY POINTS

- How is a telemedicine program created? It begins with the decision-making process to determine whether synchronous telemedicine is appropriate for the clinician and the practice. Recent COVID-19 changes are also discussed.
- Web presence is discussed, with a brief tutorial and high-impact tips to ensure an effective virtual visit.
- Various models of synchronous telemedicine to consider are explored, including center-to-center and center-to-home models.
- Technical considerations are reviewed. These considerations change rapidly, and telemedicine models adapt to an ever-changing market where the traditional office visit is being challenged by direct-to-consumer models.
- Population health: telemedicine and artificial intelligence–assisted algorithms may allow high-level overview of large patient populations to address sleep concerns as they relate to population health, occupational medicine, and transportation safety.

IS TELEMEDICINE APPROPRIATE?

When entertaining the idea of telemedicine, the first step is to assess whether this type of clinical visit is appropriate for the clinician and the clinical practice. The American Academy of Sleep Medicine (AASM) released a position statement on the use of sleep telemedicine in 2015 and this may help clinicians who are contemplating adding sleep telemedicine to their practice. Part of this assessment includes an honest evaluation of the clinician's comfort level both with pursuing something new and with technology itself. If the clinician is initially apprehensive about either one, it is often helpful to identify the specific issues that lead to the discomfort. For example, the clinician may be intimidated by the software or the hardware required to perform a synchronous telemedicine encounter. There are classes available in person or online that may ease this discomfort. The clinician should consider being coached or trained by someone with technical expertise. Perhaps the clinician is concerned about learning how to use an examination extender, such as an electronic stethoscope, and how to coordinate a physical examination with a telepresenter. Often there are educational resources provided by the vendor with a support team who can provide troubleshooting tips. The better the source of the discomfort can be identified, the more likely it is that a specific resolution exists. Is the

* ND Center for Sleep, 103B 4152 30th Avenue South Fargo, ND 58104, USA
E-mail address: skhosla@medbridgegroup.com

Sleep Med Clin 15 (2020) 347–358
https://doi.org/10.1016/j.jsmc.2020.05.002
1556-407X/20/© 2020 Elsevier Inc. All rights reserved.

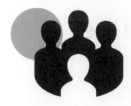

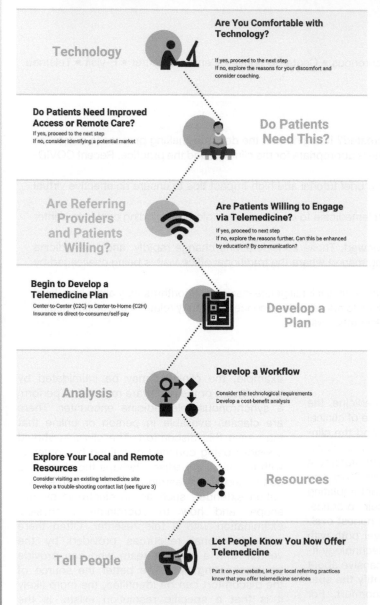

Fig. 1. Algorithm to determine whether telemedicine is appropriate for a practice. (*Courtesy of* Dr Barry Fields, Atlanta, GA.)

clinician uncomfortable with the idea of engaging with a patient remotely? There are classes and blogs available to teach about Web-side manner, such as this Webinar created by the National Consortium of Telehealth Resource Centers (https://youtu.be/IpF9gW9OZQQ). An algorithm to consider following is provided in **Fig. 1**.

Once the clinician has become more comfortable with the idea of telemedicine, the second step is to objectively look at the clinic workflow. Is it already overbooked? How long is the patient wait time? If the practice is currently overwhelmed with patients, then realistically there is no room for telemedicine patients. If the clinician is planning to transition current in-person patients to a telemedicine model, or if it has been determined that there is room in the clinic schedule, the next step is to assess the financial feasibility of a telemedicine practice.

This assessment involves an evaluation of both fixed costs (eg, start-up costs) and recurring costs (monthly costs). These costs depend on the level of sophistication of the system. If there is a geographic area that will be served, a determination needs to be made regarding telemedicine versus establishing a satellite clinic. A sample cost analysis worksheet is provided in **Tables 1–3**.

An important consideration is whether or not Medicare will reimburse for the remote visits. This consideration has recently changed with the COVID-19 pandemic. Because it is unclear whether current reimbursement guidelines will continue, this article includes some resources in case regulations revert back to the pre-COVID-19 situation. A helpful Web site is http://datawarehouse.hrsa.gov/telehealthAdvisor/telehealthEligibility.aspx, which is based on the geographic location of the originating site (where the patient is). Once these fields have been populated and totals tabulated, a fiscal decision needs to be made regarding the feasibility of a telemedicine practice. If this makes financial sense for the practice, it is time to involve the clinical staff. The next step requires an objective look at the staff. Will they be champions or will they create barriers?

The staff's attitude toward telemedicine is critical. It is important to include them in the decision-making process. Telemedicine may initially seem like a way to streamline the clinic personnel but, in reality, the staff will have shifting responsibilities. A nurse will still be needed to room the patient and obtain vital signs. The scheduling staff will need to schedule telemedicine visits, unless a platform that will automate this process is used. The information technology (IT) staff will need to be involved in the telemedicine setup. They will need to ensure a Health Insurance Portability and Accountability Act (HIPAA)–compliant visit that satisfies the regulatory aspects of telemedicine. They are all already part of the team but now will likely work more closely on the telemedicine project. When staff members recognize the value of telemedicine, they often instinctively become telemedicine champions, especially when they see how patients benefit from this technology. It is vital to discuss the intent with the team and assess their willingness to embrace synchronous telemedicine. Listen to and acknowledge their concerns. A successful telemedicine program requires the support of the team. As Dr Singh points out earlier in this issue, synchronous telemedicine is an audiovisual, real-time visit between the patient and provider. As such, the staff need to treat this as any other clinic visit including previsit and postvisit duties. The aim of a telemedicine visit is to mirror the in-person visit as much as possible. If there is paperwork that needs to be completed before the visit, the same will need to be completed before a telemedicine visit. This requirement also applies to documentation after

Table 1				
Cost analysis worksheet for monthly costs				
	Item	C2H ($)	C2C ($)	Satellite ($)
Monthly costs	Clinic space	NA	–_____	–_____
	Telemedicine technician/presenter	NA	–_____	NA
	Other staff	NA	–_____	–_____
	Practitioner travel	NA	NA	–_____
	Staff travel	NA	NA	–_____
	Software platform	–_____	–_____	NA
	Public awareness/advertising	–_____	–_____	–_____
	Lost new in-person visits at primary clinic	–_____	–_____	–_____
	Lost follow-up in-person visits at primary clinic	–_____	–_____	–_____
	Lost HSATs from primary clinic	–_____	–_____	–_____
	Lost PSGs from primary clinic	–_____	–_____	–_____
—	Other	–_____	–_____	–_____
—	Total monthly costs	–_____	–_____	–_____

Abbreviation: NA, not applicable.
Courtesy of Dr Barry Fields, Atlanta, GA.

Table 2
Cost analysis worksheet for single costs (start-up costs)

	Item	C2H Telemedicine ($)	C2C Telemedicine ($)	Satellite Clinic ($)
Single costs	Web camera	–_____	–_____	NA
	Telestethoscope	NA	–_____	NA
	Oral examination camera	NA	–_____	NA
	Other	–_____	–_____	–_____
Total single costs		–_____	–_____	–_____

Courtesy of Dr Barry Fields, Atlanta, GA.

the visit and checkout procedures, including scheduling a test or arranging for Durable Medical Equipment (DME).

The next consideration is with respect to the potential patients. Will they be amenable to a telemedicine visit? Some patients are rapid adopters of technology; others are more reluctant. Will the patients be willing to be seen via telemedicine? In our telemedicine practice, we initially assumed, as did many others, that younger patients would be more amenable to telemedicine visits.[1] We were surprised that our patient population had a bimodal distribution. We had many younger patients but also had a significant number of older patients who were of retirement age. It is important to recognize that this group of patients grew up with a television in the home. They are pleased with their electronic tablets. They are comfortable engaging in a telemedicine encounter.[2] In our experience, they were very satisfied with a telemedicine clinic offering. As the investigators of this study[2] noted, telemedicine brings medicine back to the narrative description of the presenting complaint (History of Present Illness) and the clinician's observational skills. The ability to communicate with a patient is an essential skill necessary for a successful telemedicine encounter. Providers need to show that they are listening to their patients to help earn their trust. This study concluded that telemedicine was more reminiscent of traditional doctor-patient interactions that relied more on communication and trust rather than primarily depending on test results.

WHAT ARE THE DIFFERENT TELEMEDICINE MODELS?

Synchronous telemedicine can be performed in several ways. The 2 major models are center-to-center (C2C) and center-to-home (C2H).

C2C requires the patient to be seen in an approved clinical location.[3] This location may be the primary care physician's office, the dental office,[4] or in some states the school.[5] There are trained personnel who will greet the patient, set up the telemedicine visit for the patient, and take vital signs and appropriate clinical history. This process is similar to an in-person visit and current previsit duties performed by the nurse or medical assistant. There is someone available if there are any issues that arise during the visit. The health care practitioner conducting the telemedicine visit is physically in the practitioner's own clinic. The patient is physically at a health care facility (originating site) that is closer to the patient's home. This arrangement reduces travel time for the patient. This type of visit is recognized by many insurance payors and most states have parity for these visits,[3] which means that the reimbursement for a telemedicine visit must be the same as for an in-person visit as mandated by state legislation, although there are nuances in this legislation and variances between states.

C2H allows the patient to be seen in a nonclinical setting, such as the home or place of work. There are no trained personnel with the patient and the patient navigates through the telemedicine

Table 3
Cost analysis worksheet final tally

	C2H Telemedicine	C2C Telemedicine	Satellite Clinic
Total revenue	+_____	+_____	+_____
Total single costs	–_____	–_____	–_____
Total monthly costs	–_____	–_____	–_____
Net gain/loss	_____	_____	_____

Courtesy of Barry Fields. Atlanta, GA.

visit alone. Many telemedicine platforms offer immediate assistance in case of technical issues and the platforms are usually straightforward and uncomplicated. These visits have historically not been covered by insurance payors; however, with the national emergency created by COVID-19, these visits are now being reimbursed by most payors. With the 1135 waiver, C2H telemedicine has suddenly become mainstream. At the time of this writing, readily available audiovideo platforms such as Skype and FaceTime are able to be used. It is unclear whether reimbursement will continue after the coronavirus emergency. It is also unclear whether these platforms will continue to be accepted. Realistically, an HIPAA-compliant model will need to emerge.

The C2H model has been gaining popularity among the direct-to-consumer models for several years. These models are typically hosted by a telemedicine platform company. Patients pay for this directly. Fees are paid to the health care practitioner with part of the fee going to the telemedicine company. Sometimes these fees are submitted to insurance companies by the patient or they are taken out of a health-savings account. Data show that patients are willing to pay for this convenience.[6,7]

There has also been a shift toward e-visits in health care systems as well as with certain insurance carriers.[8] These e-visits are hosted on the insurance company's Web site or on the Web site for a hospital system. Insurance coverage for these visits is variable and often depends on the specific plan.[9] Health care systems seem to be moving toward interchangeable in-person and telemedicine visits with consistent providers,[10] and this has long been a criticism of telemedicine. There have been a few companies who have offered virtual visits with mostly out-of-state physicians using a direct-to-consumer model, which did not always allow for longitudinal care and often directly opposed primary care models, although not universally. Data show that patients prefer to be seen by their own providers via telemedicine than a new provider via telemedicine, even if that new provider is within the same health system.[11] By larger health systems offering electronic visits with their own providers, patients benefit from a shared electronic health record as well as continuity of care. They are able to schedule a visit online, upload relevant information or paperwork, and engage in a telemedicine visit with their own health team from their home or place of work. These visits are now routinely performed during the COVID-19 pandemic and costs have either been waived or covered under payor policies. Some differences in these two models are outlined in **Fig. 2**.

There are also 2 models of scheduling patients. If staff are traveling to the patient location (originating site) and using dedicated equipment (such as a telemedicine robot or telemedicine cart that is the property of the practice), it may be prudent to devote the entire day to that particular site. This approach allows higher efficiency because staff are traveling to set up the equipment and serve as the telepresenter.

If staff are shared with the originating site, it is then feasible to place those patients into existing clinic slots (any day) that are more convenient for the patients. It is then possible to quickly switch from in-person visits to virtual visits, which is particularly helpful if the telemedicine platform being used is Web based with plug-and-play equipment such as the camera, e-stethoscope, speakers, and microphone that remain at the originating site. This model is often used when starting out with a telemedicine practice because the financial outlay is significantly lower. This model can also be used for the direct-to-consumer C2H telemedicine model (minus the e-stethoscope), although some clinicians prefer to have a dedicated day for these patients as well. By incorporating virtual visits with in-person visits, any patient no-show can potentially be filled by a virtual last-minute visit.[12] Many telemedicine

Telemedicine Model	Center to Home (C2H)	Center to Center (C2C)
Advantages	• Implementation costs lower • Ease of patient access • Patients familiar with own technology	• More similar to live office visit • Utilization of personnel and diagnostic tools • Reliable and higher-quality technology
Disadvantages	• Privacy more difficult to control • No tools or personnel available • Variable signal quality/reliability	• Remote site agreement required • Higher equipment and personnel costs • Less convenient to patients

Fig. 2. Comparison of C2H versus C2C models. (*Courtesy of* Dr. Jaspal Singh, Charlotte, NC.)

platforms allow providers to toggle their availability in real time so patients can connect immediately.

TECHNICAL CONSIDERATIONS

The most basic requirements for a telemedicine visit are a video camera, a microphone, and a high-speed Internet connection. The telemedicine platform must provide a secure connection. The technology has improved so rapidly that the minimum standards can be satisfied with a typical smartphone or tablet device,[13] although authentication may be required[14] for security. There are no current HIPAA requirements for smartphone authentication, but this is likely to be updated.[15]

One important consideration is the telemedicine platform itself, which must be a secure, HIPAA-compliant private connection. Recently, these requirements have been loosened under the 1135 national emergency waiver but will likely revert back to requiring a HIPAA-compliant system. The specific platform largely depends on the clinician's preference. There are companies that offer monthly subscriptions and supply all of the necessary training. Some interface with the existing electronic medical record (EMR). The features offered vary. Some include the ability to take notes and generate a PDF of the visit that can be directly uploaded into the EMR. Some include the ability to take credit card information from the patient before the visit and provide billing services. Some submit billing to insurance for reimbursement. The levels of service are variable and are apparent in the cost structure.

If the clinical visit will require more than the minimal technology, there are varying levels of sophistication available for telemedicine. There is a telemedicine robot[16] that can be manipulated remotely to maneuver through clinic hallways. This robot has a video camera, microphone, and screen. Often there are drawers that can be opened in order to use examination extenders, such as an electronic stethoscope or oral camera. These can be placed into position by the telepresenter or by the patient with the clinician's guidance. The sounds are transmitted through the software and audio system. There is often the ability to record these sounds and place them into the health record, although there is little reason to do so. Because this is not routinely done with an in-person visit, there is no compelling reason to do this for a telemedicine visit. The purpose of the telemedicine visit is to mirror the in-person visit. If it is something that would not be routinely done in person, there is likely no reason to do it during a telemedicine visit.

Examination extenders are also available without a telemedicine robot. They are add-on pieces of equipment that either plug into the computer (usually via USB port) or are stand-alone devices with internal power and memory. There are oral cameras[17] that send the image via the video connection directly. These images can be shared with the patient or seen by the provider alone. These images can be saved into the electronic health record if so desired (ie, preoperative evaluation for adenotonsillectomy or to share images with a consultant; eg, a dentist for oral appliance therapy [OAT]). These more robust technologies carry a higher price tag but, depending on the practice, many prove to be invaluable. Choosing hardware and software that interface with the current system may be wise. Communicate with the IT staff, as well as the administrators and fellow clinicians, to determine the most realistic setup for the practice.

It is often helpful to create a telemedicine troubleshooting contact list. This list is a quick reference containing contact information for IT support, the originating site (where the patient is), the Internet provider, and (most importantly) the telepresenter's contact information. It is vital to be able to reach the telepresenter throughout the patient visit in case there are technical issues or if there are clinical issues requiring immediate intervention. The information should also be readily available for the telepresenter, and a similar troubleshooting contact list should be available at the originating site. These lists are often physically placed beside the computer monitor for easy access or are adhered to the monitor itself. They should be updated on a regular basis as part of the telemedicine policy guidelines. A sample troubleshooting contact list is provided in **Fig. 3**.

WHAT ARE THE LEGAL IMPLICATIONS?

This brief article is not meant to be a comprehensive legal review. Clinicians should consult their attorneys because this article is not intended to be legal advice.

According to the American Telemedicine Association,[18] a synchronous telemedicine visit is perfectly legal as long as clinicians abide by official guidelines. These guidelines vary from state to state. Some important considerations before implementing a telemedicine practice revolve around these issues:

1. Can a doctor-patient relationship be established via telemedicine?
2. Can medications be prescribed for patients seen via telemedicine?

Troubleshooting Contact List

As you are setting up your telemedicine program, make sure to fill out the troubleshooting contact list, so you are prepared in case issues arise.

Local Coordinator:

Contact Name:_____

Telephone Number:_____ (ext):_____

Email:_____

Remote Site Coordinator:

Contact Name:_____

Telephone Number:_____ (ext):_____

Email:_____

Telepresenter:

Contact Name:_____

Telephone Number:_____ (ext):_____

Email:_____

Hardware Issues

General Information Technology Help Desk: (*Local Computer Issues*)

Contact Name:_____

Telephone Number:_____ (ext):_____

Email:_____

Computer make, model, serial number:_ _____

Internet Service Provider: (*Networking Issues*)

Contact Name:_____

Telephone Number:_____ (ext):_____

Email _____

Fig. 3. Sample telemedicine troubleshooting contact list. (*From* AASM Sleep Technology Implementation Guide, American Academy of Sleep Medicine Telemedicine Implementation Task Force, 2016, Jaspal Singh, MD Chair; M. Safwan Badr, MD; Lawrence Epstein, MD; Barry Fields, MD; Dennis Hwang, MD; Seema Khosla, MD; Kimberly Mims, MD; Brandon Peters, MD; Afifa Shamim-Uzzaman, MD; Emerson Wickwire; with permission.)

3. Can testing be ordered for patients seen via telemedicine?
4. Can DME treatment be prescribed for patients seen via telemedicine, including positive airway pressure (PAP), OAT, and nasal expiratory PAP devices?

The answers to these specific questions depend on the state. Telemedicine is patient-centric. The rules apply to the state where the patient is, but health care practitioners must also be in compliance with their home state regulations regarding the practice of telemedicine. This requirement is a little simpler for practices where the provider and the patient are in the same state, which is often a good place to begin. The Interstate Medical Licensure Compact[19] has continued to grow and helps to streamline the application process if multiple state licenses are desired. It is not a national license but aims to remove barriers and share information to facilitate licensure in multiple states.

There are also nuances to these legal questions. For example, in states where a doctor-patient relationship cannot be established via telemedicine, clinicians are often able to provide telemedicine services to the established patients. It is common, in these circumstances, for the initial visit to take place in person with all of the follow-up done via telemedicine. This situation is also an excellent opportunity to query the patients on their willingness to engage in follow-up telemedicine visits. This would satisfy Centers for Medicare & Medicaid Services (CMS) regulations[20] regarding the physical examination, which must be documented in order to script PAP therapy (body mass index, neck circumference, focused cardiopulmonary and upper airway system evaluation).[21]

WILL THE CLINICIAN GET PAID FOR A TELEMEDICINE VISIT?

No matter how altruistic the clinicians' intentions, a telemedicine practice cannot survive if telemedicine visits are not reimbursed. Billing for a telemedicine visit is straightforward but must be done correctly. The visit is billed with a typical Evaluation and Management (E&M) code for professional services along with a telemedicine modifier code.[22] The telemedicine modifier is GT Q3014. GT indicates that the synchronous telemedicine occurred via interactive audio and video. The video component must be present. CMS (Centers for Medicare and Medicaid Services) asks for a 95 modifier to be used instead. There is a GQ code, which indicates that the service was asynchronous. As of January 2020, there were only 16 states that did not recognize synchronous telemedicine visits.[23] It is also important to note that, during the 1135 COVID-19 waiver, these modifiers are changing rapidly with significant differences between payors. It is vital to check with local payors to ensure appropriate payment for services.

Telemedicine visits between a clinician and a patient must mirror the in-person visit. The billing also mirrors billing for an in-person visit. Billing can be done for time or via a traditional E&M code plus a GT modifier. It is important to recognize that this is not a reduced fee modifier. Synchronous telemedicine visits are reimbursed at the same rate as the in-person visit in most states[24] where parity legislation has been passed. There is also a facility fee that can be charged in addition to the E&M code. Although this facility fee is not always reimbursed, when it is, it also allows the clinician to recoup expenses for telemedicine equipment and/or room rental at the originating site. Billing is the critical component of a telemedicine practice; if this part is not executed correctly, the practice will not survive. Billing and reimbursement are discussed elsewhere in this issue.

HOW TO PERFORM A TELEMEDICINE VISIT

The emphasis thus far has been to show that telemedicine is not a new way of practicing medicine, it is simply a tool that allows the practice of medicine remotely. The patient visit is the same, with few exceptions. The history taking is the same, and the laboratory review and decision-making processes are the same. However, the differences are important to recognize. It is vital to take the time to create an appropriate clinical experience for both the patient and the clinician, which involves setting up the environment and paying attention to specific details that will allow the clinician to execute a successful telemedicine encounter. These details are outlined in **Fig. 4**.

1. Be mindful of the clinical environment. This requirement pertains mostly to the C2C model, where the patient's surroundings can be controlled. Although this is also important in the C2H model, the clinician has less control over the patient's space. Before the C2H visit, educational, assistive materials should be provided to the patient to ensure a private, quiet room with good lighting and minimal disruptions. The same requirement applies to the C2C visit. It should be treated the same as an in-person visit. The telepresenter should ensure that the door is closed and that there are no distractions (eg, loud noises, frequent disruptions, conversations in the hallway) during the visit. Privacy should be ensured and patients treated in a professional manner.

2. Pay attention to the details. The space should be well lit for both the patient and the clinician. It is helpful to do a trial run before the visit to ensure that the audio and video are of good quality ahead of time.

3. Be mindful of the equipment. The audiovisual equipment should be positioned unobtrusively. The microphone should be placed in close proximity to the patient. The speakers should be adjusted to a comfortable level. The patient should be able to quickly forget about the equipment as the visit continues.

4. Pay attention to the eyeline. Maintaining eye contact is an important part of any clinic visit. Patients often think that clinicians are not paying attention if they are not maintaining eye contact throughout the visit.[25] This requirement is much easier to do in person than via a virtual visit. It is therefore important for clinicians to be mindful of where their eyes appear to be looking. It is helpful at the beginning of the visit for clinicians to assure their patients that they are looking at them on the monitor but that they may have to avert their eyes in order to take notes. It is worthwhile to have the telepresenter sit in the patient's seat before the visit to provide feedback about the eye position. Pay attention to both the horizontal and the vertical eyelines. Once the telepresenter has confirmed where the eyes should be, place a marker on the screen to serve as a reminder of where to look. If picture in picture is available on the platform, it is helpful to move the thumbnail view into that location so as to be able to quickly look the patient in the eye while also making sure that the expression is appropriate and conveys engagement in the visit.

5. Minimize the e-mail and turn off phone notifications. This session is a patient interaction that mirrors the in-person interaction. Clinicians do not check e-mails during visits

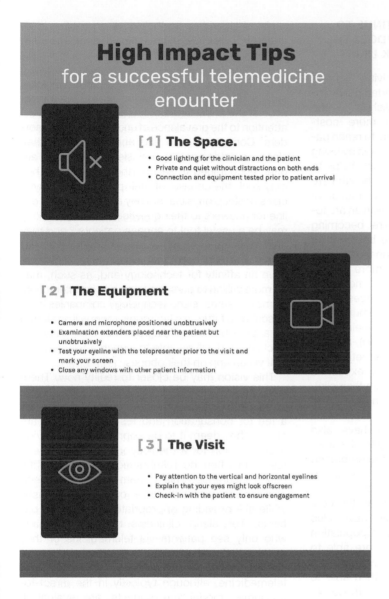

High Impact Tips
for a successful telemedicine enounter

[1] The Space.
- Good lighting for the clinician and the patient
- Private and quiet without distractions on both ends
- Connection and equipment tested prior to patient arrival

[2] The Equipment
- Camera and microphone positioned unobtrusively
- Examination extenders placed near the patient but unobtrusively
- Test your eyeline with the telepresenter prior to the visit and mark your screen
- Close any windows with other patient information

[3] The Visit
- Pay attention to the vertical and horizontal eyelines
- Explain that your eyes might look offscreen
- Check-in with the patient to ensure engagement

Fig. 4. High-impact tips for a successful telemedicine encounter.

when a patient is in the office and they should not check them during an e-visit.

6. Prepare ahead of time. Test the connection. Check the lighting and the sound. Make sure the telemedicine platform is functioning appropriately, including the screen-share feature.

7. Ensure that no other patient information is on the computer if the intention is to share the screen; this is another reason why e-mails should be turned off or minimized with notifications turned off.

8. Clinicians can choose which of the monitors to share. It is often helpful to move the specific information related to the patient to the external monitor and then share that screen with the patient. This ability allows clinicians to then have the EMR pulled up on the primary monitor. They can then move the selected documents that they wish to share.

9. Clinicians may wish to have the patient upload information before the visit, such as sleep logs or sleep tracker information. They can also complete the regular paperwork ahead of time and upload this information for the review.

10. Above all, remember that a telemedicine visit is a regular patient visit that is done remotely. Relax. Once the clinician has practiced and worked out the details, it should flow the same way as the regular in-person clinic visits.

HOW WILL TELEMEDICINE CONTINUE TO CHANGE THE PRACTICE? WHAT DOES THE FUTURE OF TELEMEDICINE LOOK LIKE?

Clinical algorithms respond to evolving technology. What used to require fully attended polysomnography can now be accomplished in the patient's home faster and in a more cost-effective manner.[26] Clinicians are able to reach patients who would otherwise never be seen by using telemedicine technology.[27] This, in turn, helps to keep communities healthier and keep health care dollars within those communities. The practice of sleep medicine continues to change with an arc toward patient-centricity. Patients are becoming health care consumers. Health care has evolved from a paternalistic approach to one of shared decision making. Patients expect more convenience[28] and this often results in more on-demand knowledge (patients can access their electronic health records), faster communication (they can communicate directly with their health care practitioners via secure messaging), and access to new information (via the Internet). Many of these health care consumers also expect to be able to have a face-to-face visit with their clinicians on demand in the convenience of their homes or places of work. Telemedicine has become an expectation.[29] Studies have also shown that patients are willing to pay for this convenience.[6,30,31] Many companies have embraced a direct-to-consumer approach, as described earlier in relation to telemedicine models.

Health care systems have also seen the cost savings of telemedicine.[32,33] They have also been able to apply this technology to population health management. Large systems are able to mine their data and identify patients who are at a high risk of sleep apnea. They are then able to deploy questionnaires and engage with those patients. Those patients are then evaluated by a clinician, either via questionnaire or an e-visit. Testing is ordered and the results are reviewed by the overseeing physician. Treatment can be ordered and follow-up is also done via telemedicine. By managing large populations, health care systems can improve the overall health of their covered entities. This ability results in a reduction in health care spending, which can then benefit the system as a whole.[34] Artificial intelligence (AI)–assisted algorithms can be applied to the electronic health record to further evaluate which patients may be appropriate for further evaluation and testing/treatment.[35] As the electronic health record and AI both improve, this may become standard for large health systems or those who are self-insured. Insurance companies may also apply AI-assisted algorithms to their covered entities in an attempt to reduce overall health care spending by identifying patients at high risk.

Much more patient-initiated testing is now being done. The ubiquity of consumer sleep technology, such as fitness trackers, has increased the awareness of the importance of sleep. It has also drawn attention to the prevalence of underlying sleep disorders. Consumers who find abnormalities in their sleep, as determined by their sleep technology, are often encouraged to seek further evaluation. They may seek the counsel of their primary care physicians or sleep physicians. They are also looking online for answers to their questions. This technology may be a useful tool to engage patients[36] and may allow patients to be more aware of their sleep. Patients who use consumer sleep technology may have an affinity for technology and, as such, may be more willing to pursue a telemedicine interaction. Some consumer sleep technology companies have described a future in which consumers will be alerted to a possible sleep disorder via their wearable trackers, and will be able to launch a telemedicine visit via an app on their phones.[37]

This vision may be closer to reality now. There are several tele–sleep clinics that currently operate using the direct-to-consumer model. They charge a fee for consultation and testing, and then are able, if they deem it to be appropriate, to provide a prescription for a medication or device. These fees can often be reimbursed by the patient's health insurance. This system allows tele–sleep clinicians to work with lower operating expenses while still providing appropriate care to their patients. Tele-sleep clinicians may be clinicians who only see patients via telemedicine or they may be clinicians who also see patients in person. Longitudinal relationships can be maintained via telemedicine, although typically in the direct-to-consumer model the patients are evaluated, treated, and then sent back to their primary care physicians. If issues arise, they can reconsult the tele–sleep clinician but usually these relationships are episodic. For patients with straightforward obstructive sleep apnea (OSA) who do well on PAP therapy, this model works well.

Implementing a telemedicine program may seem daunting. It is important to recognize that telemedicine is simply another method of delivering medical care. It is not a new way to practice medicine; clinicians are able to practice medicine as they currently do, but it allows them to connect with their patients using technology. This technology allows clinicians to expand their current reach and, more importantly, allows them to reach patients who may not have ever been seen because of geographic or travel limitations.[38] Technology helps clinicians to deliver care into areas that are underserved. By providing health care to these populations, the overall health of the communities improves.[38]

Sleep medicine suffers from a lack of urgency. When people have chest pain, they recognize that they need to go to the emergency room (ER) to be seen. There are public service announcements teaching about the signs and symptoms of a stroke so people can identify it sooner and seek treatment more quickly. Very few people go to the ER to be evaluated for snoring. The current model of OSA diagnosis leaves 80% of patients undiagnosed.[39] This system is extremely fragmented with numerous bottlenecks along the algorithm. One common barrier is the need to travel to be seen by a sleep specialist, particularly in rural communities. This situation creates yet another barrier to care. Untreated sleep disorders carry with them significant morbidity.[40] Clearly, the current paradigm is far from ideal. Telemedicine is one way to reduce barriers for patients. By eliminating the need for them to travel great distances, they are more likely to undergo testing and treatment of their underlying sleep disorders. Consumer sleep technology may be another way to identify those at higher risk of a sleep disorder. Those consumers may then pursue further evaluation and treatment. AI algorithms applied to large populations may identify more patients at high risk of a sleep disorder. Perhaps all of these modalities will help clinicians to improve their ability to identify and treat the immense number of patients who have an undiagnosed and therefore untreated sleep disorder.

Telemedicine is just another tool in the toolkit. It is up to clinicians to decide how they want to use this technology to reach their patients before nonclinicians make those decisions instead. Embracing this technology, which has been around for decades, may allow the gaps in the current health care algorithm at last to be bridged. The COVID-19 pandemic has been an ignition event for telemedicine. Now is the time to embrace this technology and build a sustainable telemedicine program.

DISCLOSURE

The author has nothing to disclose.

REFERENCES

1. Available at: https://www.beckershospitalreview.com/healthcare-information-technology/82-of-young-adults-would-prefer-telehealth-to-in-person-visit.html Accessed January 19, 2020.
2. Available at: https://www.ncbi.nlm.nih.gov/pmc/articles/PMC5752645/ Accessed January 19, 2020.
3. Center for connected health policy. Available at: https://www.cchpca.org. Accessed January 19, 2020.
4. Available at: https://mhealthintelligence.com/news/dentists-use-telehealth-to-improve-access-to-care-and-fight-a-phobia Accessed January 19, 2020.
5. Available at: https://www.amdtelemedicine.com/telemedicine-resources/documents/ATAstate-medicaid-best-practice—school-based-telehealth.pdf Accessed January 19, 2020.
6. Available at: https://patientengagementhit.com/news/77-of-patients-want-access-to-virtual-care-telehealth Accessed January 19, 2020.
7. Available at: https://www.idigitalhealth.com/news/patients-clinicians-satisfied-with-telehealth-for-followup-care Accessed January 19, 2020.
8. Available at: https://www.bcbsmonlinevisits.com/landing.htm Accessed January 19, 2020.
9. Available at: https://www.bcbs.com/the-health-of-america/articles/telehealth-quality-care-your-fingertips Accessed January 19, 2020.
10. Available at: https://www.advisory.com/research/care-transformation-center/care-transformation-center-blog/2018/10/behavioral-health-access Accessed January 19, 2020.
11. Available at: https://www.ncbi.nlm.nih.gov/pmc/articles/PMC5704580/ Accessed January 19, 2020.
12. Available at: https://blog.evisit.com/telemedicine-solves-costly-problem-no-shows Accessed January 19, 2020.
13. Gough F, Budhrani S, Cohn E, et al. Practice guidelines for live, on demand primary and urgent care. Telemed J E Health 2015;21:233–41.
14. Available at: https://www.ncbi.nlm.nih.gov/pmc/articles/PMC5716614/ Accessed January 19, 2020.
15. Luxton DD, Kayl R, Mishkind MC. mHealth data security: the need for HIPAA-compliant standardization. Telemed J E Health 2012;18:284–8. https://doi.org/10.1089/tmj.2011.0180. Available at:.
16. Available at: https://www.businesswire.com/news/home/20130506005495/en/InTouch-Health-iRobot-Announce-Customers-Install-RP-VITATM Accessed January 19, 2020.
17. Available at: https://fireflyglobal.com/de605-general-examination-camera/. Accessed January 19, 2020.
18. Available at: https://www.cchpca.org/telehealth-policy/current-state-laws-and-reimbursement-policies Accessed January 19, 2020.
19. Available at: https://imlcc.org/ Accessed January 19, 2020.
20. Available at: https://www.genesishealth.com/care-treatment/neuroscience/sleep/patient-resources/medicare-guidelines-for-cpap/ Accessed January 19, 2020.
21. Available at: https://www.usa.philips.com/c-dam/b2bhc/master/whitepapers/sleep-therapy-compliance/1084892_PhysDocumentforPAP_HelpHint.pdf Accessed January 19, 2020.
22. Available at: https://liveclinic.com/blog/gt-modifier-telemedicine-billing Accessed January 19, 2020.

23. Available at: https://www.americantelemed.org/initiatives/2019-state-of-the-states-report-coverage-and-reimbursement/ Accessed January 19, 2020.

24. Available at: https://www.americantelemed.org/policy/state-activity/ Accessed January 19, 2020.

25. Available at: https://www.physicianspractice.com/pearls/patients-three-biggest-complaints-about-your-practice Accessed January 19, 2020.

26. He K, Kim R, Kapur VK. Home- vs. Laboratory-based management of OSA: an economic review. Curr Sleep Med Rep 2016;2:107–13.

27. Available at: https://www.cdc.gov/chronicdisease/resources/publications/factsheets/telehealth-in-rural-communities.htm Accessed January 19, 2020.

28. Available at: https://www.ortholive.com/blog/but-do-patients-want-telehealth-the-survey-says-yes Accessed January 19, 2020.

29. Available at: https://patientengagementhit.com/news/retail-consumer-experience-key-in-consumer-driven-healthcare Accessed January 19, 2020.

30. Available at: https://www.ncbi.nlm.nih.gov/pubmed/15603629 Accessed January 19, 2020.

31. Available at: https://www.prnewswire.com/news-releases/virtual-visits-with-medical-specialists-draw-strong-consumer-demand-survey-shows-300475757.html Accessed January 19, 2020.

32. Available at: https://www.urac.org/blog/telehealth-offers-cost-savings-opportunities-hospitals-and-patients Accessed January 19, 2020.

33. Available at: https://www.healthcarefinancenews.com/news/telehealth-eliminates-time-and-distance-save-money Accessed January 19, 2020.

34. Available at: https://mhealthintelligence.com/news/healthcare-wakes-up-to-the-value-of-mhealth-and-sleep Accessed January 19, 2020.

35. Available at: https://link.springer.com/article/10.1007/s41649-019-00096-0.

36. Khosla S, Deak MC, Gault D, et al. Consumer sleep technology: an American Academy of Sleep Medicine position statement. J Clin Sleep Med 2018; 14(5):877–80.

37. Connor Heneghan, PhD, speaker at the AASM Sleep Disruptors Conference, Chicago, March 2019.

38. Available at: https://www.cdc.gov/chronicdisease/pdf/factsheets/Rural-Health-Telehealth-H.pdf Accessed January 19, 2020.

39. Available at: https://aasm.org/resources/pdf/sleep-apnea-economic-crisis.pdf Accessed January 19, 2020.

40. Available at: https://www.sleephealth.org/sleephealth/the-state-of-sleephealth-in-america/ Accessed January 19, 2020.

Telehealth, Telemedicine, and Obstructive Sleep Apnea

Sharon Schutte-Rodin, MD, DABSM, CBSM

KEYWORDS

- Telehealth • Telemedicine • Telemonitoring • Remote patient monitoring (RPM)
- Obstructive sleep apnea (OSA) • Electronic health record (EHR)
- Patient-reported outcomes (PROs) • e-consult

KEY POINTS

- Obstructive sleep apnea (OSA) telehealth options may be used to replace or supplement none, some, or all steps in the evaluation, testing, treatments, and management of OSA. All telehealth steps must adhere to best-practice and quality-measure OSA guidelines.
- OSA telehealth pathways may be adapted for continuous positive airway pressure (CPAP) and non-CPAP treatments.
- Not all patients may be appropriate for 1 common OSA telemanagement pathway. If considering 1 standardized OSA telehealth path, prior evaluation for other sleep breathing, sleep, and medical disorders and comorbidities is needed because these patients may require different telepathways.
- OSA telemanagement may improve communications, workflows, outcomes, patient satisfaction, costs, and e-data collection. E-data collection enhances uses for individual and group analytics, phenotyping, testing and treatment selections, high-risk identification and targeted support, and comparative and multispecialty therapy studies.
- Clinical and consumer sleep and medical technology advancements, deep learning and artificial intelligence algorithms, and the roles of insurers, pharmacies, and Web services will continue to change the evolving landscape of OSA telemanagement.

DEFINITIONS: TELEHEALTH, TELEMEDICINE, AND UNCOMPLICATED OBSTRUCTIVE SLEEP APNEA

There is no 1 definition for either telehealth or telemedicine. There also are a variety of teleservices and e-services. Simply stated, adding tele to the front of a word indicates distant and adding e in front of a word indicates electronic.[1] A broader construct, telehealth, is not a specific service. Telehealth "is a collection of means or methods for enhancing health care, public health, and health education delivery and support using telecommunication technologies."[2] Using the definitions of telehealth and telemedicine similarly, the American Telemedicine Association (ATA) defines telemedicine as "the remote delivery of health care services and clinical information using telecommunications technology."[3] Having the most narrow telehealth definition but with impact of the economic feasibility of incorporating OSA telehealth into clinical practice workflows, the definition by the Centers for Medicare and Medicaid Services (CMS) relates to payment to providers for specific telehealth clinical services.[4] These telehealth applications include live (synchronous) videoconferencing, store-and-forward (asynchronous) videoconferencing, remote patient monitoring, and mobile health (mHealth).[5] As the definition associated

Penn Sleep Center, 3624 Market Street, 2nd Floor, Philadelphia, PA 19104, USA
E-mail address: Sharon.Schutte-Rodin@pennmedicine.upenn.edu

Sleep Med Clin 15 (2020) 359–375
https://doi.org/10.1016/j.jsmc.2020.05.003
1556-407X/20/© 2020 Elsevier Inc. All rights reserved.

with payment by CMS and some private insurers, this may be the definition affecting providers when choosing e-technology in practice workflows. In the context of the management of obstructive sleep apnea (OSA), revisiting definitions of telehealth and telemedicine assists OSA clinicians in choosing teleapplications that may be most useful to their practice workflows and available resources.

This article focuses on the broader, more inclusive, telehealth definitions for the evaluation, diagnosis, treatment, and chronic management of OSA (**Fig. 1**). Further, although the evaluation of OSA includes the ability to recognize central sleep apnea and other respiratory breathing and sleep disorders, this article addresses the uses of telehealth specifically for uncomplicated OSA. When considering standard OSA telehealth pathways and options for a patient, it is of critical importance to screen and evaluate for other sleep breathing disorders and related comorbidities because these would require different telehealth management. Ideally, clinicians use unique telehealth pathways using validated preselection algorithms for different patient OSA phenotypes and comorbidities. An interim simplified strategy to identity uncomplicated OSA for standard OSA telehealth

care may be similar to the evaluation used when choosing attended polysomnography (PSG) versus unattended home sleep apnea testing (HSAT) for uncomplicated adult OSA.[6–9]

Many sleep medicine clinicians worldwide have been practicing forms of OSA telehealth for decades (such as remote online study interpretations, e-communications, and remote continuous positive airway pressure [CPAP] data monitoring). Likewise, many patients with OSA have been participating in e-care and self-education (eg, online interactive CPAP applications such as MyAir or DreamMapper), with their positive airway pressure (PAP) home medical equipment (HME) companies (using calls, texts, emails, PAP unit messaging), and with providers through EHR message portals.[10–13]

Because the landscape for provider payment of teleservices is rapidly changing and varies from state to state and country to country, OSA providers should be aware of local payments for teleservices.[4,5,14,15] In addition to enhancing and expanding OSA care, providers may find that the integration and implementation of teleservices into daily OSA workflows may realize valuable indirect workflow savings and patient satisfaction benefits.[11,16–21] Recognizing the importance of

Definitions: Telehealth, Telemedicine, Uncomplicated Obstructive Sleep Apnea

OSA Telehealth Implementation: Standardized e-Care Within OSA Best Practice and Quality Measures

OSA Evaluation and Telehealth
Baseline Tele-evaluation Options
Hub-and-spoke Model and E-consults

OSA Diagnosis and Telehealth
OSA Tele-testing
E-Communications of Test Results, OSA Severity, and Treatments
Data Analytics for Testing and Treatment Paths

OSA Treatments and Telehealth

CPAP Tele-management
CPAP: Remote Education and Set-up
CPAP Telemonitoring
Reviewing Remote CPAP Data
Long-term Remote CPAP Data Monitoring

Non-CPAP Device Tele-management
Other Non-CPAP Remote Device Monitoring

Other Telehealth Chronic OSA Management (All treatments)

Discussion

Fig. 1. Article outline.

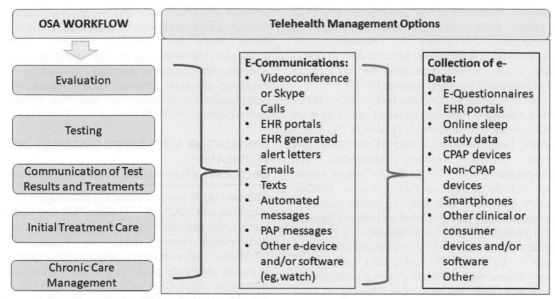

Fig. 2. OSA workflows and telemanagement options. CPAP, continuous PAP.

using sleep telemedicine tools, the American Academy of Sleep Medicine (AASM) launched the SleepTM Web site and provided additional resources (Singh 2015, Implementation Guide, AASM Web site) to assist clinicians with the integration and implementation of telemedicine into sleep practices.[14,22,23]

OBSTRUCTIVE SLEEP APNEA TELEHEALTH: IMPLEMENTATION OF STANDARDIZED E-CARE WITHIN OBSTRUCTIVE SLEEP APNEA BEST-PRACTICE GUIDELINES AND AMERICAN ACADEMY OF SLEEP MEDICINE QUALITY MEASURES

Whether delivered in person or using telehealth technologies, the evaluation, diagnosis, treatment, and chronic management of OSA must be delivered at the same best-practice level using accepted standards of care, quality measures, and guidelines.[6–9,22,24–34] Although clinical care standards for telemedicine should mirror those of in-person visits, OSA telecare and e-care also open opportunities to expand new ways to deliver improved OSA care access, between-visit care, communications, education, cost savings, individual and big data access, and monitoring quality-measure outcomes data.[11,16,17,19–22,35–51] Moreover, in addition to providing a structure for traditional OSA care, the guidelines allow for customized variations in telehealth care implementation using available local practice (technical, staff, financial) resources, regional insurance coverages, and societal best-practice guidelines. This strength provides flexibility

for using e-care in none, some, or many of the steps in OSA evaluation, diagnosis, and management. This framework and associated teleopportunities and e-opportunities for OSA care are described in more detail later.

A traditional OSA workflow may include the clinical evaluation, testing, communication of the diagnosis and treatment options with the patient, initial treatment care, and chronic care management. While keeping within OSA best-practice and quality-measure guidelines and the OSA provider's current workflow and resources, there are numerous opportunities for teleservices and e-services to replace, supplement, provide additional interim care and education, or improve practice workflows and costs for each of the OSA treatments (**Fig. 2**). Although many telehealth studies focus on CPAP treatment and outcomes, telehealth applications for other OSA treatments, chronic management strategies, and big-data deep learning applications may be realized.

OBSTRUCTIVE SLEEP APNEA EVALUATION AND TELEHEALTH
Baseline Tele-evaluation Options

Patients with OSA enter sleep-center workflows through varied pathways. Before testing and diagnosis, patients initially may be evaluated by the primary care physician (PCP), by sleep medicine or other specialists, or by self-referral.[22,25,52,53] Thus, identification of possible comorbid apnea conditions and risks during the evaluation and before testing is important in the selection of any OSA workflow path, test type selection, treatment choice, and follow-up care.[6–8,54] Telehealth e-tools and e-consults offer added opportunities to document screening and evaluation for appropriate OSA telehealth uses and management.[22,23,35]

For OSA, whether done at a face-to-face visit or using telehealth options, baseline and follow-up OSA symptoms, sleepiness, quality of life (QoL), weight, blood pressure, comorbid disorders, and motor vehicle accident assessment are documented.[22,24,26,29,55] Evaluation e-tool examples include patient-reported outcomes (PROs), quality measures, and sleep symptom questionnaires that may be completed by patients through EHR patient portals, sleep middleware or other medical or consumer OSA risk assessment software, or by phone.[56,57] Cukor and colleagues[57] used phone call OSA educational dialogue to show improved likelihood of scheduling an OSA evaluation in a black community sample. Moreover, consumer sleep technologies and digital health tools continue to advance from entertainment to validated sleep and physiologic collection devices.[58–60] Alerted by feedback about sleep questionnaire completion, snoring, heart rate variations, and/or sleep disruption, consumers may collect increasingly valuable apnea-related symptom data to share in the apnea evaluation process either as an individual self-referral or through computer algorithm risk identification and device alerts.[61,62] Likewise, whether done at a face-to-face visit or using telehealth options (such as video or blood pressure/weight telecollection), baseline and follow-up blood pressure and weight assessments with appropriate counseling are performed.[26,30,58,63–66]

Hub-and-Spoke Model and E-consults

Sarmiento and colleagues[42] provide a concise summary of the Veterans' Affairs (VA) TeleSleep hub-and-spoke model of (synchronous) video teleconferencing and Remote Veteran Apnea Management Platform (REVAMP), a VA web-application which allows veterans to complete PRO questionnaires, communicate with providers, use online self-help tutorials, and view CPAP data. REVAMP providers either review the PRO and electronic health record (EHR) information during the televisit or provide an (asynchronous) e-consult determination to proceed directly to HSAT testing (without the televisit). Later, test results, CPAP prescriptions, and modem data are incorporated in the EHR for further telemanagement. E-consults also are gaining use outside of the VA system, particularly when providers are practicing

within 1 EHR.[67,68] Although e-consults improve access, costs, and time to diagnosis and treatment, there are reported concerns about increased PCP workload, unpaid time for provider and practice support services, ownership of follow-up services, potential liability issues, and unanticipated consequences such as missed comorbidities.[18,53,67–70]

OBSTRUCTIVE SLEEP APNEA DIAGNOSIS AND TELEHEATH
Obstructive Sleep Apnea Teletesting Options

PSG and HSAT provide accepted pathways for the diagnosis of OSA.[6–9,28,31,71] Both PSG and HSAT commonly use forms of (asynchronous store-and-forward) remote data review.[22] Of note, HSAT and consumer device technologies continue to evolve and undergo direct gold standard and/or outcomes-based OSA validation testing to further expand telehealth testing options.[50,72–77] Several wearables with pulse oximetry Spo_2, heart rate variability, actigraphy, and deep learning algorithms are currently under US Food and Drug Administration (FDA) evaluation as HSAT-type devices.[78] Further, ongoing HSAT validation studies for specific subgroups of at-risk patients continue to expand possible HSAT telehealth services. Saletu and colleagues[76] described the use of HSAT OSA diagnosis for inpatient rehabilitation of cerebrovascular accident, Kauta and colleagues[79] described the use of inpatient HSAT and PAP therapy reducing 30-day readmission rates, and Choi and colleagues[80] reported the use of Watch-PAT for adolescent OSA diagnosis. Although the use of autoCPAP for high-risk patients with OSA without formal testing has been proposed, the exclusion of comorbidities (such as obesity hypoventilation), lack of OSA severity assessment, validated preselection algorithms for patient phenotypes and comorbidity exclusions, and inconclusive correlation with low autoCPAP pressures currently preclude treatment of patients without any OSA testing and severity assessment.[6,24,27,30,81,82]

E-communications of Test Results, Obstructive Sleep Apnea Severity, and Treatment Options

In keeping with OSA best-practice and quality-measure guidelines, the communications of the test results, OSA severity, and treatment options with patients may be done at face-to-face visits or using e-communications such as videoconferencing, phone, EHR portal messaging, Skype, or other e-communications.[21,35,42,44,45,50] Education of OSA risks, test results, treatment options, sleepiness and driving, and weight and blood pressure monitoring may be supplemented with video links, Web sites, and other e-communication formats.[8,22,24,35,44] With respect to the e-communication of test results on OSA telehealth outcomes, there is considerable variation in who provides the test results to patients in many telehealth studies. Test results may be e-communicated to patients by sleep medicine or other physicians, nurses, nurse practitioners, physician assistants, laboratory technicians, respiratory therapists, home equipment therapists, or other trained staff.[20–22,39,42,44–46,49,52,83] Teasing out the use of only e-communication of test results on treatment outcomes is further confounded by OSA telehealth studies using different telecommunication forms as well as different timing for the e-evaluation, PAP adherence monitoring, and PAP e-support combined with the e-communication of the test results.[84] Nevertheless, many OSA telehealth studies and reviews include combinations of e-visits for e-communication of test results, some type of adherence telemonitoring, and CPAP support e-communications, which are discussed later.[11,19–22,35–38,40–51,85,86]

Data Analytics for Testing and Treatment Paths

In addition to clinical guidelines for OSA test type and promising OSA testing technologies, deep learning and artificial intelligence models using phenotyping, EHR data, and/or other consumer or medical sensor devices and applications may provide insights for OSA risk assessment and test prioritization, choosing the optimum test type, or selection of personalized treatment paths.[87–96] Stretch and colleagues[87] proposed a machine learning model to predict patients having nondiagnostic HSATs and requiring PSG, whereas Mencar and colleagues[97] and Huang and colleagues[92,93] suggested models to predict OSA severity risk for testing prioritization. Using HL-7 integration of software or internal EHR portals, PRO and sleep questionnaire data within EHRs may allow the interface of comorbid and other clinical EHR big data to further enhance identification of OSA risk, phenotypes, optimum test type, and outcomes.[56,98]

OBSTRUCTIVE SLEEP APNEA TREATMENTS AND TELEHEALTH

Current recommended OSA treatment options include PAP, positional apnea devices, oral appliances, and upper airway surgeries.[8,24,26–28,30,31,99,100] Adjunct OSA management includes, but is not limited to, weight loss;

HME and PAP device patient engagement technologies; cognitive behavior therapy for insomnia (CBT-I) with comorbid insomnia; and the use of supportive education, coaching, monitoring, and management e-communications.[22,30,44–47,86,101]

CONTINUOUS POSITIVE AIRWAY PRESSURE TELEMANAGEMENT
Continuous Positive Airway Pressure: Remote Education and Setup

For patients who receive CPAP as initial therapy, a PAP Rx often is sent from the provider (EHR) to an HME for either face-to-face, group class, Skype, or videoconference remote CPAP setup and education.[35,36,42,45,47,49,50,85] For appropriate patients, the use of autoCPAP allows the Rx to be in either fixed or auto-Rx modes and also permits flexibility in resetting the Rx remotely through online pressure adjustments as clinically needed.[27,30] Initial education and mask choice by sleep technicians or HME therapists is thought to influence early compliance but is recognized to be labor intensive, particularly if done in person in the patient's home. When adhering to AASM telemedicine standards, both remote education and video CPAP setups may offer decreased labor time while maintaining equivalent or improved CPAP compliance and satisfaction.[22] Close relationships and monitoring of HMEs by providers are key in minimizing setup errors and ensuring telemonitoring protocols.[102] Mask fitting facial recognition software, use of mask sizers (during video or Skype setups), mask fit packs (containing several cushion sizes), and deep learning analysis of mask fitting selection phenotypes may expand remote CPAP mask selection and setup options.[103–105]

Using e-questionnaires, insurance and clinical EHR data, and phenotyping models, patients at high risk for nonadherence might receive added or targeted tele-educational and support protocols such as adjunct CBT-I with comorbid insomnia.[86,96,101,104,106,107] Although early educational interventions before CPAP initiation are strongly recommended and behavioral and troubleshooting interventions are suggested, specific standard or tele-education formats are not mandated.[30] This noted, the effect of tele-education alone on compliance overall does not seem robust,[45] which may be because of confounding factors such as the variability of the initial and following tele-education deliveries, as well as easy availability of Internet sites and industry-sponsored Web OSA and CPAP educational resources for patients with OSA. Kuna and colleagues,[108] Malhotra and colleagues,[109] Hostler and colleagues,[12] Hardy and colleagues,[10] Lynch and colleagues,[110] and Shaughnessy and colleagues[111] found improved compliance for patients given Web access to their data and companion educational resources. Isetta and colleagues[85,112] and Fields and colleagues[21] reported improved compliance and satisfaction with videoconference training. Parikh and colleagues[20] showed similar compliance and patient satisfaction with videoconferencing compared with standard visit care. Hwang and colleagues[45] explored the use of telemedicine OSA education (teled) and automated compliance messaging and found that teled alone did not increase adherence, but teled did improve clinic attendance and further increased compliance in the automated messaging group. For patients identified as being at risk for poor CPAP compliance, Guralnick and colleagues[113] noted that educational videos did not improve compliance or clinic show rates.

Continuous Positive Airway Pressure Telemonitoring

Numerous studies have shown similar or increased CPAP compliance with various forms of CPAP data telemonitoring, which may include automated message data alerts, coaching and reinforcement emails/texts/calls/EHR messages/online educational and motivational support, and Skype or videoconferencing.[11,37–39,41,43–46,48,114,115] Turino and colleagues[38] showed similar compliance with telemonitoring but improved patient satisfaction and cost savings. Murase and colleagues[51] proposed that telemedicine may assist adherence even with users for more than 3 months. Nilius and colleagues[116] and Kotzian and colleagues[117] showed improved compliance of patients with strokes with proactive telemonitoring. Further, telemonitoring of CPAP data may enable early identification of central sleep apnea/Cheyne-Stokes and congestive heart failure/cardiac disease occurrence or progression.[46,118] Tung and colleagues[118] followed 2912 patients over 5 years and found central sleep apnea and Cheyne-Stokes to be a predictor of incident atrial fibrillation.

As noted earlier, many patients are empowered to improve adherence with Web access to CPAP use, leak, and residual apnea-hypopnea index (AHI) data as well as access to online support tools.[12,13,43,44,88,108,109,111] Self-monitoring of blood pressure and weight is gaining interest. Although limited to a 4-month trial, Mendelson and colleagues[119] showed the feasibility of patient entry of blood pressure, CPAP use, sleepiness, and QoL data into smartphones for clinician review. McManus and colleagues[58] reported that patient self-monitoring of blood pressure, with or without telemonitoring, decreased blood pressure after 12 months. Personal patient cost savings have been shown to improve medication adherence, suggesting that telecare without copays also may improve adherence.[120] Likewise, HMEs are using CPAP vendor telemonitoring software such as ResMed's U-Sleep and Philips Patient Adherence Monitoring Service to improve initial CPAP compliance.[121,122]

Reviewing Remote Continuous Positive Airway Pressure Data

Sleep providers are familiar with CPAP remote data monitoring, which often focuses on initial CPAP adherence. However, the presence of significant air leak may confound the interpretation of CPAP use time, residual AHI data, and minimum/maximum/average autoCPAP pressure data. Remote data interpretation and clinical caution are indicated if an acceptable air seal is not first confirmed. Note that leak data are not included in adherence reporting in many studies. The choice of the date range also affects interpretation of remote data monitoring. For example, normal data for the past averaged 3 or 6 or 12 months may not represent recent normal or abnormal data over the past weeks. In addition, definitions and algorithms for leak, AHI, and use times may vary between CPAP unit brands.[123,124] Spo_2 monitoring is available to add separately or directly into some home CPAP unit brands, but typically Spo_2 monitoring is not part of standard OSA CPAP data monitoring. For patients empirically set up with autoCPAP, Koivumaki and colleagues[125] suggested oximetry as part of CPAP initiation of patients with baseline Spo_2 less than 92% or body mass index greater than 30 kg/m^2. Further, users may overlook that CPAP unit residual AHI is based on recording time and may include snoring and vibration in the total residual event calculations (ie, CPAP AHI is not equal to PSG AHI).[126,127] Nonetheless, CPAP remote data monitoring improves CPAP adherence and outcomes and is standard care for CPAP management.[30,33]

Long-Term Remote Continuous Positive Airway Pressure Data Monitoring

After the initial 90 days, some HMEs may decrease remote data monitoring of CPAP adherence. In a review, Murphie and colleagues[36] found variability in the frequency of long-term PAP visit or call follow-up. Telehealth offers increased care access options. However, office staff telemonitoring of voluminous nightly data from entire practices of patients is daunting and generally not reimbursable. Ideally, patients are, and continue to be, engaged in self-monitoring of Web-based data and are instructed to notify providers with changes in leak, residual AHI, use times, or clinical problems. The use of vendor software notice applications, EHR applications, middleware algorithms, and automated data alert messaging may provide a feasible solution for practices attempting to manage huge amounts of nightly CPAP data for PAP patients over years.[44,88] Using Health Level 7 (HL7) integrated PAP data within the EHR, Tan and colleagues[128] showed how an EHR could be used as the workhorse to identify real-time, abnormal PAP data on a quarterly or scheduled basis, and then send EHR-generated alert e-messages (to seek follow-up) to a large practice of clinic patients with OSA with abnormal PAP data.

OBSTRUCTIVE SLEEP APNEA TELEMANAGEMENT OF NON–CONTINUOUS POSITIVE AIRWAY PRESSURE TREATMENTS
Other Non–continuous Positive Airway Pressure Remote Device Monitoring

Although not as commercially available to patients as online CPAP data access, data alerts, and education, telemonitoring of other OSA therapy data seems to be forthcoming. Positional OSA (POSA) devices are an OSA treatment option that has more recent telemonitoring capabilities.[129–133] Although there remain discussions on definitions, subclassifications, and associated use guidelines for POSA, new technologies are allowing sleep position and compliance e-monitoring capabilities.[129–131,134–136] The addition of remote POSA adherence data to PRO and EHR data allows clearer outcomes analytics and also the valuable dimension of comparative therapy studies.[134,136,137] Similar to CPAP teleapplications, some POSA devices are FDA cleared; may be combined with other therapies; and offer online educational resources, data access, and downloadable reports to share with sleep clinicians.[132,133]

Abilities to telemonitor oral appliance (OA) compliance data are evolving. Although not yet as common as online CPAP and some POSA device data access, the use of temperature-sensing data chips embedded in the OA have provided objective OA adherence data in studies.[136–141] Commercially available SomnoDent OA uses patented software, temperature sensor, and triple axis accelerometer technologies that allow patients to upload OA use times and supine/nonsupine data for Web report access.[140] The use of OA compliance data with PRO, EHR, and AHI study data allows comparative treatment studies,

quality-measure and outcomes analysis, and prediction models.[136,137,140] Expansion of online software for OA therapy data access seems the next logical step toward OA telemanagement. In addition, like POSA and other non-CPAP therapies, such OA adherence telemonitoring would require supplemental, periodic OSA reassessment long term and as clinically indicated.[32,138,142] The American Academy of Dental Medicine recommends at least annual OA therapy follow-up.[143]

Using an implantable pulse generator and stimulation and sensing leads, hypoglossal nerve stimulation (HGNS) offers the promise of expanded future telemanagement applications. Remembering how CPAP data were originally downloaded using cards to software, HGNS compliance data currently are available using cloud-based reports after USB upload.[144] Marrying HGNS data with PRO, EHR, and AHI study data opens possibilities for comparative studies and for phenotyping, patient selection, outcomes, cost analysis, and prediction models.[145–149] Looking toward the future, although wireless transmission is not yet available, such telemonitoring software and workflows could be a next step in HGNS remote data telemanagement. Cardiologists are familiar with remote pacemaker data monitoring, including event documentation.[150–152] In the IN-TIME study, Husser and colleagues[150] described an analysis of pacemaker workflow for remote data collection and alert messages sent to clinics that then phone patients for clinical correlation. In addition, pacemaker technologies continue to advance. According to a January 2020 press release by Medtronic, the FDA recently approved the first leadless pacemaker for atrioventricular synchrony using accelerometer-based atrial sensing and a patented algorithm.[153]

Other Telehealth Chronic Obstructive Sleep Apnea Management (All Treatments)

Although the same telehealth evaluation, testing, diagnosis, and educational options are available for other OSA treatments, fewer studies have explored the use of telehealth for non-CPAP treatments. However, regardless of the chosen OSA treatment, the same best-practice initial and chronic OSA management are recommended.[8,24,32,99,100] In addition to long-term remote device data monitoring, chronic OSA management for all treatments includes reassessment of sleep and apnea symptoms, sleepiness, QoL, weight, and blood pressure, which may be assessed in person or using telehealth methods used during initial tele-evaluations.[8,24,154] E-communications with patients may help clinicians to standardize blood pressure and weight assessments and counseling.[66,155] Ideally, clinical and PRO data may be collected using scheduled e-questionnaires or device data and used within the EHR for individual and group monitoring, for creation of patient high-risk list follow-up, for comparative treatment studies, and for big data AASM and CMS quality measures.[64,91,97,98] Using PRO, EHR, compliance, and other e-data, benefits and comparisons with CPAP e-data have been explored. Mendelson and colleagues[119] did not find a difference in smartphone-collected blood pressures after 4 months of CPAP use. In separate OA studies, de Vries and colleagues[156,157] reported reductions of systolic and diastolic blood pressures comparable with CPAP and adherence comparable with CPAP. Cillo and colleagues[158] showed long-term QoL improvement and patient satisfaction with maxillomandibular advancement. Analyzing 5-year outcomes of HGNS, Woodson and colleagues[149] reported improvement of sleepiness, QoL, and AHI response.

Because OSA may change with aging, weight, menopause, and some medications, long-term OSA monitoring for all treatments is indicated.[159–161] Although autoCPAPs may adjust with weight changes, aging, menopause, disease progression, and changing medications and comorbidities over time, other treatments may not offer long-term permanent protection or adapting therapy coverage.[162–165] It seems reasonable to use HSAT-type testing for long-term follow-up of ongoing treatment efficacy, but the frequency of follow-up teletesting for non-CPAP therapies does not seem clear. For POSA and OA devices, ongoing remote data monitoring of adherence is needed. Sutherland and Cistulli[138] and Sato and Nakajima[142] discussed the importance of long-term monitoring of OA adherence and for late side effects.[32] In particular, because weight changes over time affect OSA management, long-term weight monitoring remains important. Wang and colleagues[166] showed a correlation between weight loss, reduction of tongue fat, and improved AHI following weight loss interventions. This correlation noted, weight gain has been observed years after weight loss surgeries, with some patients requiring surgical revisions for further weight reduction.[165,167] Thus, even with apparent initial successful resolution of OSA, such as with airway or weight loss surgeries, long-term monitoring for OSA reoccurrence or progression is warranted.[161–164]

Like the initial e-evaluation and e-testing, scheduled telehealth e-questionnaires, weight and comorbidity monitoring, and home screening or testing devices may offer an option for long-term tele–follow-up of non-CPAP OSA treatment. Moreover, with ongoing validation studies, some consumer sleep technologies are transitioning to reliably track snoring, sleep, oximetry, heart rate variability, and OSA screening. As well, deep learning algorithms and software to collect individual and group analysis of weight, blood pressure, sleepiness, and other quality-measure data for prediction models are advancing. For example, Cistulli and Sutherland[89] proposed the use of analytics of phenotype and other tools to help guide personalized OSA therapy approaches.

DISCUSSION

The execution of OSA clinical guidelines and practice standards is possible using traditional, hybrid, and telehealth OSA workflows. Face-to-face visits or telehealth applications may be inserted in 1 or more of the workflow steps for (1) evaluation pathways, (2) diagnosis pathways, (3) CPAP and non-CPAP treatments, and (4) long-term follow-up. Telehealth e-applications may be used for communications, education, and support in any or all of these steps. OSA telehealth offers the opportunities to increase patient access, between-visit care, consultant-provider-HME-patient communications and education, cost savings, testing and treatment type selections, and patient satisfaction.[21,35,42,47,49,50] In addition, e-data collection using telehealth expands possibilities for individual and group data analysis for AASM and CMS quality measures, phenotyping, outcomes, comparative studies, and deep learning predictive models for OSA evaluation, testing, treatment selection, and best-practice workflows.[45,46,90] Farré and colleagues pose[168] the question of whether all patients with OSA or particular phenotypes are better served for different aspects of telehealth options. Incorporation of OSA-related data and other EHR discrete data opens dimensions to better understand the relationships of OSA with OSA-related comorbidities, multispecialty therapies, and outcomes-driven practices.

However, the promise of expanded OSA telehealth applications is accompanied with cautious considerations. Practical implementation into clinical OSA workflows requires an understanding of local payment for teleservices as well as assessment of available investment, staff, EHR, and information technology resources. In addition, clear OSA telehealth algorithms to screen and identify appropriate patients are essential. Separate telehealth pathways need to be clarified for special populations or patients with combination breathing, sleep, medical, or comorbid disorders.

Telehealth offers flexibility in who delivers and takes ownership of initial and chronic OSA care and workflows. As previously described, telehealth applications may be used in none, some, or all of the OSA workflow steps. However, this workflow assumes that a boarded clinician is the OSA workflow supervisor and monitor. On its chronic disease HealthHUB Web site, a national pharmacy chain advertises that its HealthHUB providers may perform an OSA risk assessment, order home testing, review results and options, and prescribe CPAP and supplies.[169] Another pharmacy chain advertises sleep links and live provider video calls for sleep and chronic disease evaluation.[170] In these proposed care models, tele and electronic data sharing with clinicians seem vital in long-term OSA follow-up and management, particularly if these patients include those with unscreened comorbidities, requiring therapy changes, or requiring OSA problem solving. It also is unclear whether and how mergers of insurers, pharmacies, and retail chains will affect standard and telehealth OSA care and delivery.[171] How to best incorporate these and other new entities into best-practice standard, hybrid, and telehealth OSA workflows currently seems a moving environment.

The volumes of available OSA e-data also present questions on how best to monitor and use these huge datasets in daily practices as well as how to use them in deep learning predictive models.[91,95,172–174] Assuming the feasibility of automated machine alerts of abnormal OSA clinical or device data or high-risk groups, how frequently should e-alerts be advised and how will such alerts be handled in an expanded tele-workflow? While monitoring practice support resources as ample, Tan and colleagues[128] found that quarterly clinic EHR-generated alerts of abnormal PAP and other OSA therapy data provided adequate time for the correction of PAP issues and then time to generate new PAP (postintervention) data. Education and scheduled engagement of patients in self-monitoring of abnormal PRO, sleep, weight, blood pressure, and PAP e-data through e-communications with providers may be an option for some practices.[50,119] Moreover, evolving validation of clinical and consumer sleep-related technologies, sensors, devices/applications, and deep learning/artificial intelligence algorithms affect telehealth options and explosively increase available big datasets.[44,59,91,172,175–185] How telehealth will play a role in EHR information exchange with insurers and with Apple and Web service consumer e-data is developing.[186–189] For example, Apple's Healthkit offers wireless blood pressure cuffs for home blood pressure and heart rate data to interface with the EHR for clinician review. In addition, refill and health tips may be e-sent to the patient Apple Watch.[186] Other large health and sleep e-dataset resources available for OSA prediction models and telehealth applications include access to the National Institutes of Health Big Data to Knowledge and National Sleep Research Resource.[91,190] Although AASM has dedicated task forces for telemedicine, EHR, clinical and consumer sleep technologies, and artificial intelligence, the fast rate of technology development and e-datasets seems to continue to outpace clinical studies on how to best incorporate new OSA technologies, telehealth, and voluminous clinical and consumer daily data into clinical practice guidelines.

Revisiting the telehealth construct of "a collection of means or methods for enhancing health care, public health, and health education delivery and support using telecommunication technologies,"[2] it is clear that increasing applications of telehealth into the OSA workflow will continue to enhance and expand OSA care. Although there are potential future challenges in standard, hybrid, and telehealth OSA care options, AASM and other specialty groups have provided a framework and clear standards on best-practice clinical guidelines for OSA evaluation, diagnosis, treatment, and follow-up.[6–9,22,24–34] The use of telehealth in any of the OSA care steps requires the same level of attention to accepted standards of OSA care, quality measures, and clinical guidelines. With the ongoing development and validation of clinical and consumer sleep technologies, remote data monitoring, expansion of e-communications, and data analytics, the role of OSA telehealth applications and management will continue to evolve and expand. While maintaining best-practice standards, telehealth offers new dimensions and strengths in flexibility and enhancement of standard OSA workflows, and the promise for improved OSA care.

DISCLOSURE

The author has nothing to disclose.

REFERENCES

1. California telemedicine and eHealth center: a glossary of telemedicine and eHealth. Available at: http://www.caltrc.org/wp-content/uploads/2013/10/ctec_glossary_final.pdf. Accessed November 6, 2019.
2. Center for Connected Health Policy (The National Telehealth Policy Resource Center): What is

Telehealth?. Available at: https://www.cchpca.org/about/about-telehealth. Accessed January 26, 2020.

3. American Telemedicine Association: What is Telemedicine?. Available at: http://legacy.americantelemed.org/main/about/about-telemedicine/telemedicine-faqs. Accessed January 26, 2020.

4. Centers for Medicare and Medicaid Services (CMS) Medical Learning Network: Telehealth Service. Available at: https://www.cms.gov/Outreach-and-Education/Medicare-Learning-Network-MLN/MLNProducts/downloads/TelehealthSrvcsfctsht.pdf. Accessed November 26, 2019.

5. HealthIT.gov (Official website of the Office of the National Coordinator for Health Information Technology- ONC): ONC): Telemedicine and Telehealth. Available at: https://www.healthit.gov/topic/health-it-initiatives/telemedicine-and-telehealth. Accessed November 26, 2019.

6. Kapur VK, Auckley DH, Chowdhuri S, et al. Clinical practice guideline for diagnostic testing for adult obstructive sleep apnea: an American Academy of Sleep Medicine Clinical Practice Guideline. J Clin Sleep Med 2017;13:479–504.

7. Rosen IM, Kirsch DB, Carden KA, et al. Clinical use of a home sleep apnea test: an updated American Academy of Sleep Medicine position statement. J Clin Sleep Med 2018;14(12):2075–7.

8. Epstein LJ, Kristo D, Strollo PJ Jr, et al. Clinical guideline for the evaluation, management and long-term care of obstructive sleep apnea in adults. J Clin Sleep Med 2009;5(3):263–76.

9. Collop NA, Anderson WM, Boehlecke B, et al. Clinical guidelines for the use of unattended portable monitors in the diagnosis of obstructive sleep apnea in adult patients. Portable Monitoring Task Force of the American Academy of Sleep Medicine. J Clin Sleep Med 2007;3(7):737–47.

10. Hardy W, Powers J, Jasko JG, et al. DreamMapper white paper: a mobile application and website to engage sleep apnea patients in PAP therapy and improve adherence to treatment. Available at: http://incenter.medical.philips.com/doclib/enc/fetch/2000/4504/577242/577256/588723/588747/sleepmapper-tx-whitepaper.pdf%3fnodeid%3d11228847%26vernum%3d-2.

11. Munafo D, Hevener W, Crocker M, et al. A telehealth program for CPAP adherence reduces labor and yields similar adherence and efficacy when compared to standard of care. Sleep Breath 2016;20(2):777–85.

12. Hostler JM, Sheikh KL, Andrada TF, et al. A mobile, web-based system can improve positive airway pressure adherence. J Sleep Res 2017;26(2):139–46.

13. ResMed My Air. Available at: https://myair.resmed.com/. Accessed April 30, 2020.

14. American Academy of Sleep Medicine Clinical Resources: Telemedicine. Available at: https://aasm.org/clinical-resources/telemedicine/. Accessed January 20, 2020.

15. Telligen, gpTRAC. Telehealth: Start-Up and Resource Guide. Version 1.1. 2014. Available at: https://gptrac.org/wp-content/uploads/2015/01/TelligenTelehealthGuide-Final-2014.pdf.

16. Isetta V, Negrín M, Monasterio C, et al. A Bayesian cost-effectiveness analysis of a telemedicine-based strategy for the management of sleep apnoea: a multicentre randomised controlled trial. Thorax 2015;70(11):1054–61.

17. Russo JE, McCool RR, Davies LVA. Telemedicine: an analysis of cost and time savings. Telemed J E Health 2016;22(3):209–15.

18. Thaker DA, Monypenny R, Olver I, et al. Cost savings from a telemedicine model of care in northern Queensland, Australia. Med J Aust 2013;199:414–7.

19. Dullet NW, Geraghty EM, Kaufman T, et al. Impact of a university-based outpatient telemedicine program on time savings, travel costs, and environmental pollutants. Value Health 2017;2:542–6.

20. Parikh R, Touvelle MN, Wang H, et al. Sleep telemedicine: patient satisfaction and treatment adherence. Telemed J E Health 2011;17:609–14.

21. Fields BG, Behari PP, McCloskey S, et al. Remote ambulatory management of veterans with obstructive sleep apnea. Sleep 2016;39(3):501–9.

22. Singh J, Badr MS, Diebert W, et al. American Academy of Sleep Medicine (AASM) position paper for the use of telemedicine for the diagnosis and treatment of sleep disorders. J Clin Sleep Med 2015;11(10):1187–98.

23. Singh J, Badr MS, Epstein L, et al. Sleep telemedicine implementation guide. American Academy of Sleep Medicine; 2015. Available at: https://aasm.org/clinical-resources/telemedicine/. Accessed November 22, 2019.

24. Aurora RN, Collop NA, Jacobowitz O, et al. Quality measures for the care of adult patients with obstructive sleep apnea. J Clin Sleep Med 2015;11(3):357–83.

25. Aurora RN, Quan SF. Quality measure for screening for adult obstructive sleep apnea by primary care physicians. J Clin Sleep Med 2016;12(8):1185–7.

26. Morgenthaler TI, Aronsky AJ, Carden KA, et al. Measurement of quality to improve care in sleep medicine. J Clin Sleep Med 2015;11(3):279–91.

27. Morgenthaler TI, Aurora RN, Brown T, et al. Practice parameters for the use of autotitrating continuous positive airway pressure devices for titrating pressures and treating adult patients with obstructive sleep apnea syndrome: an update for 2007. An

American Academy of Sleep Medicine report. Sleep 2008;31(1):141–7.

28. Fleetham J, Ayas N, Bradley D, et al. Canadian Thoracic Society 2011 guideline update: diagnosis and treatment of sleep disordered breathing. Can Respir J 2011;18(1):24–47.

29. Gamaldo C, Buenaver L, Chernyshev O, et al, OSA Assessment Tools Task Force of the American Academy of Sleep Medicine. Evaluation of clinical tools to screen and assess for obstructive sleep apnea. J Clin Sleep Med 2018;14(7):1239–44.

30. Patil SP, Ayappa IA, Caples SM, et al. Treatment of adult obstructive sleep apnea with positive airway pressure: an American Academy of Sleep Medicine clinical practice guideline. J Clin Sleep Med 2019;15(2):335–43.

31. Qaseem A, Holty J, Owens D, et al. Management of obstructive sleep apnea in adults: a clinical practice guideline from the American College of Physicians. Ann Intern Med 2013;159(7):471–83.

32. Ramar K, Dort LC, Katz SG, et al. Clinical practice guideline for the treatment of obstructive sleep apnea and snoring with oral appliance therapy: an update for 2015. J Clin Sleep Med 2015;11(7): 773–827.

33. Schwab RJ, Badr SM, Epstein LJ, et al. An official American Thoracic Society statement: continuous positive airway pressure adherence tracking systems. The optimal monitoring strategies and outcome measures in adults. Am J Respir Crit Care Med 2013;188:613–20.

34. Kushida CA, Littner MR, Morgenthaler T, et al. Practice parameters for the indications for polysomnography and related procedures: an update for 2005. Sleep 2005;28:499–521.

35. Bruyneel M. Telemedicine in the diagnosis and treatment of sleep apnoea. Eur Respir Rev 2019; 28:180093.

36. Murphie P, Little S, Paton R, et al. Defining the core components of a clinical review of people using continuous positive airway pressure therapy to treat obstructive sleep apnea: an international e-Delphi study. J Clin Sleep Med 2018;14(10): 1679–87.

37. Hoet F, Libert W, Sanida C, et al. Telemonitoring in continuous positive airway pressure-treated patients improves delay to first intervention and early compliance: a randomized trial. Sleep Med 2017; 39:77–83, 26(2):139-146.

38. Turino C, de Batlle J, Woehrle H, et al. Management of continuous positive airway pressure treatment compliance using telemonitoring in obstructive sleep apnoea. Eur Respir J 2017;49:1601128.

39. Smith CE, Dauz ER, Clements F, et al. Telehealth services to improve nonadherence: a placebo-controlled study. Telemed J E Health 2006;12: 289–96.

40. Smith I, Nadig V, Lasserson TJ. Educational, supportive and behavioural interventions to improve usage of continuous positive airway pressure machines for adults with obstructive sleep apnoea. Cochrane Database Syst Rev 2009;(2):CD007736.

41. Sparrow D, Aloia M, Demolles DA, et al. A telemedicine intervention to improve adherence to continuous positive airway pressure: a randomised controlled trial. Thorax 2010;65:1061–6.

42. Sarmiento KF, Folmer RL, Stepnowsky CJ, et al. National expansion of sleep telemedicine for veterans: the telesleep program. J Clin Sleep Med 2019; 15(9):1355–64.

43. Schoch OD, Baty F, Boesch M, et al. Telemedicine for continuous positive airway pressure in sleep apnea. A randomized, controlled study. Ann Am Thorac Soc 2019;16(12):1550–7.

44. Hwang D. Monitoring progress and adherence with positive airway pressure therapy for obstructive sleep apnea: the roles of telemedicine and mobile health applications. Sleep Med Clin 2016;11:161–71.

45. Hwang D, Chang JW, Benjafield AV, et al. Effect of telemedicine education and telemonitoring on continuous positive airway pressure adherence. The Tele-OSA randomized trial. Am J Respir Crit Care Med 2018;197(1):117–26.

46. Pepin JL, Tamisier R, Hwang D, et al. Does remote monitoring change OSA management and CPAP adherence? Respirology 2017;22(8):1508–17.

47. Suarez-Giron M, Bonsignore MR, Montserrat JM. New organisation for follow-up and assessment of treatment efficacy in sleep apnoea. Eur Respir Rev 2019;28:190059.

48. Fox N, Hirsch-Allen A, Goodfellow E, et al. The impact of a telemedicine monitoring system on positive airway pressure adherence in patients with obstructive sleep apnea: a randomized controlled trial. Sleep 2012;35(4):477–81.

49. Lugo VM, Garmendia O, Suarez-Girón M, et al. Comprehensive management of obstructive sleep apnea by telemedicine: clinical improvement and cost-effectiveness of a Virtual Sleep Unit. A randomized controlled trial. PLoS One 2019;14(10): e0224069.

50. Villanueva JA, Suarez MC, Garmendia O, et al. The role of telemedicine and mobile health in the monitoring of sleep-breathing disorders: improving patient outcomes. Smart Homecare Technology TeleHealth 2017;4:1–11.

51. Murase K, Tanizawa K, Minami T, et al. A randomized controlled trial of telemedicine for long-term sleep apnea CPAP management. Ann Am Thorac Soc 2019. https://doi.org/10.1513/AnnalsATS.201907-494OC.

52. Chai-Coetzer CL, Antic NA, Rowland LS, et al. Primary care vs specialist sleep center management of obstructive sleep apnea and daytime sleepiness

and quality of life: a randomized trial. JAMA 2013; 309(10):997–1004.

53. Osman MA, Schick-Makaroff K, Thompson S, et al. Barriers and facilitators for implementation of electronic consultations (eConsult) to enhance access to specialist care: a scoping review. BMJ Glob Health 2019;4(5):e001629.

54. Mokhlesi B, Masa JF, Brozek JL, et al. Evaluation and management of obesity hypoventilation syndrome. An official American Thoracic Society Clinical Practice Guideline. Am J Respir Crit Care Med 2019;200(3):e6–24.

55. Ibáñez V, Silva J, Cauli O. A survey on sleep assessment methods. PeerJ 2018;6:e4849.

56. Chang Y, Staley B, Simonsen S, et al. Transitioning from paper to electronic health record collection of Epworth sleepiness scale (ESS) for quality measures. Sleep 2018;41(1):404.

57. Cukor D, Pencille M, Ver Halen N, et al. An RCT comparing remotely delivered adherence promotion for sleep apnea assessment against an information control in a black community sample. Sleep Health 2018;4(4):369–76.

58. McManus RJ, Mant J, Franssen M, et al. Efficacy of self-monitored blood pressure, with or without telemonitoring, for titration of antihypertensive medication (TASMINH4): an unmasked randomised controlled trial. Lancet 2018;391(10124):949–59.

59. Consumer Technology Association and Heart Rhythm Society. Guidance for wearable health solutions white paper. 2020. Available at: https://shop.cta.tech/products/guidance-for-wearable-health-solutions. Accessed January 26, 2020.

60. Dias D, Paulo Silva Cunha J. Wearable health devices—vital sign monitoring, systems and technologies. Sensors 2018;18(8):2414.

61. Katyayan A, Yadav V, Mishra P, et al. Computer algorithms in assessment of obstructive sleep apnoea syndrome and its application in estimating prevalence of sleep related disorders in population. Indian J Otolaryngol Head Neck Surg 2019; 71(3):352–9.

62. Turakhia M, Perez M, Desai M, et al. Results of a large-scale, app-based study to identify atrial fibrillation using a smartwatch: the Apple Heart Study. Presented at the 68th American College of Cardiology Scientific Session, New Orleans, Louisiana; March 16–18, 2019. Abstract 19-LB-20253.

63. Rifkin DE, Abdelmalek JA, Miraclev CM, et al. Linking clinic and home: a randomized, controlled clinical effectiveness trial of real-time, wireless blood pressure monitoring for older patients with kidney disease and hypertension. Blood Press Monit 2013;18(1):8–15.

64. Margolis KL, Asche SE, Dehmer SP, et al. Long-term outcomes of the effects of home blood pressure telemonitoring and pharmacist management on blood pressure among adults with uncontrolled hypertension: follow-up of a cluster randomized clinical trial. JAMA Netw Open 2018;1(5): e181617.

65. Houser SH, Joseph R, Puro N, et al. Use of technology in the management of obesity: a literature review. Perspect Health Inf Manag 2019;16(Fall):1c.

66. Casey DE, Thomas RJ, Bhalla V, et al. 2019 AHA/ACC clinical performance and quality measures for adults with high blood pressure: a report of the American College of Cardiology/American Heart Association Task Force on Performance Measures. Circ Cardiovasc Qual Outcomes 2019;12:e000057.

67. Deeds SA, Dowdell KJ, Chew LD, et al. Implementing an Opt-in eConsult program at seven academic medical centers: a qualitative analysis of primary care provider experiences. J Gen Intern Med 2019;34(8):1427–33.

68. Kent J. How eConsults could transform care coordination and access. In: mHealth Intelligence. 2019. Available at: https://mhealthintelligence.com/news/how-econsults-could-transform-care-coordination-and-access. Accessed November 18, 2019.

69. Lee MS, Ray KN, Mehrotra A, et al. Primary care practitioners' perceptions of electronic consult systems: a qualitative analysis. JAMA Intern Med 2018;178(6):782–9.

70. Vimalananda VG, Gupte G, Seraj SM, et al. Electronic consultations (e-consults) to improve access to specialty care: a systematic review and narrative synthesis. J Telemed Telecare 2015;21(6):323–30.

71. Kuna ST, Gurubhagavatula I, Maislin G, et al. Non-inferiority of functional outcome in ambulatory management of obstructive sleep apnea. Am J Respir Crit Care Med 2011;183(9):1238–44.

72. Sands SA, Owens RL, Malhotra A. New approaches to diagnosing sleep-disordered breathing. Sleep Med Clin 2016;11(2):143–52.

73. Yalamanchali S, Farajian V, Hamilton C, et al. Diagnosis of obstructive sleep apnea by peripheral arterial tonometry: meta-analysis. JAMA Otolaryngol Head Neck Surg 2013;139(12):1343–50.

74. Watson NF, Lawlor C, Raymann RJ. Will consumer sleep technologies change the way we practice sleep medicine? J Clin Sleep Med 2019;15(1): 159–61.

75. Khosla S, Deak MC, Gault D, et al. Consumer sleep technology: an American Academy of Sleep Medicine position statement. J Clin Sleep Med 2018; 14(5):877–80.

76. Saletu MT, Kotzian ST, Schwarzinger A, et al. Home sleep apnea testing is a feasible and accurate method to diagnose obstructive sleep apnea in stroke patients during in-hospital rehabilitation. J Clin Sleep Med 2018;14(9):1495–501.

77. Penzel T, Schöbel C, Fietze I. New technology to assess sleep apnea: wearables, smartphones, and

accessories [version 1; peer review: 2 approved]. F1000Res 2018;7(F1000 Faculty Rev):413.

78. American Academy of sleep medicine clinical resources for #SleepTechnology. Available at: https://aasm.org/consumer-clinical-sleep-technology/. Accessed January 20, 2020.

79. Kauta SR, Keenan BT, Goldberg L, et al. Diagnosis and treatment of sleep disordered breathing in hospitalized cardiac patients: a reduction in 30-day hospital readmission rates. J Clin Sleep Med 2014;10(10):1051–9.

80. Choi JH, Lee B, Lee JY, et al. Validating the Watch-PAT for diagnosing obstructive sleep apnea in adolescents. J Clin Sleep Med 2018;14(10):1741–7.

81. Nigro CA, Borsini E, Dibur E, et al. Indication of CPAP without a sleep study in patients with high pretest probability of Obstructive Sleep Apnea. Sleep Breath 2019. https://doi.org/10.1007/s11325-019-01949-6.

82. Drummond F, Doelken P, Ahmed QA, et al. Empiric auto-titrating CPAP in people with suspected obstructive sleep apnea. J Clin Sleep Med 2010; 6(2):140–5.

83. Parthasarathy S, Subramanian S, Quan SF. A multicenter prospective comparative effectiveness study of the effect of physician certification and center accreditation on patient-centered outcomes in obstructive sleep apnea. J Clin Sleep Med 2014;10:243–9.

84. Pamidi S, Knutson KL, Ghods F, et al. The impact of sleep consultation prior to a diagnostic polysomnogram on continuous positive airway pressure adherence. Chest 2012;141:51–7.

85. Isetta V, Negrín MA, Monasterio C, et al. A Bayesian cost-effectiveness analysis of a telemedicine-based strategy for the management of sleep apnoea: a multicentre randomised controlled trial. Thorax 2015;70(11):1054–61.

86. Wozniak DR, Lasserson TJ, Smith I. Educational, supportive and behavioural interventions to improve usage of continuous positive airway pressure machines in adults with obstructive sleep apnoea. Cochrane Database Syst Rev 2014;(1): CD007736.

87. Stretch R, Ryden A, Fung CH, et al. Predicting non-diagnostic home sleep apnea tests using machine learning. J Clin Sleep Med 2019;15(11):1599–608.

88. Cistulli PA, Armistead J, Pepin JL, et al. Short-term CPAP adherence in obstructive sleep apnea: a big data analysis using real world data. Sleep Med 2019;59:114–6.

89. Cistulli PA, Sutherland K. Phenotyping obstructive sleep apnoea- bringing precision oral appliance therapy. J Oral Rehabil 2019;46:1185–91.

90. Mostafa SS, Mendonça F, Ravelo-García AG, et al. A systematic review of detecting sleep apnea using deep learning. Sensors (Basel) 2019; 19(22). https://doi.org/10.3390/s19224934.

91. Budhiraja R, Thomas R, Kim M, et al. The role of big data in the management of sleep-disordered breathing. Sleep Med Clin 2016;11:241–55.

92. Huang W, Lee P, Liu Y, et al. 0495 prediction of obstructive sleep apnea using machine learning technique. Sleep 2018;41(S1):A186.

93. Huang W-C, Lee P-L, Liu Y, et al. Support vector machine prediction of obstructive sleep apnea in a large-scale Chinese clinical sample. Sleep 2020; zsz295. https://doi.org/10.1093/sleep/zsz295.

94. Bates DW, Saria S, Ohno-Machado L, et al. Big data in health care: using analytics to identify and manage high-risk and high-cost patients. Health Aff 2014;33(7):1123–31.

95. Liu Y, Chen PC, Krause J, et al. How to read articles that use machine learning: users' guides to the medical literature. JAMA 2019;322(18):1806–16.

96. Sunwoo BY, Light M, Malhotra A. Strategies to augment adherence in the management of sleep-disordered breathing. Respirology 2020;25:363–71.

97. Mencar C, Gallo C, Mantero, et al. Application of machine learning to predict obstructive sleep apnea syndrome (OSAS) severity. Health Inform J 2019. https://doi.org/10.1177/1460458218824725.

98. Staley B, Keenan BT, Simonsen S, et al. Using an Electronic Health Record (EHR) to collect and use quality-of-life data for AASM process and outcomes quality measures. Sleep 2018;41(1):402.

99. Aurora RN, Casey KR, Kristo D, et al. Practice parameters for the surgical modifications of the upper airway for obstructive sleep apnea in adults. Sleep 2010;33(10):1408–13.

100. Morgenthaler TI, Kapen S, Lee-Chiong T, et al. Practice parameters for the medical therapy of obstructive sleep apnea. Sleep 2006;29(8):1031–5.

101. Sweetman A, Lack L, Catcheside PG, et al. Cognitive and behavioral therapy for insomnia increases the use of continuous positive airway pressure therapy in obstructive sleep apnea participants with comorbid insomnia: a randomized clinical trial. Sleep 2019;42(12) [pii:zsz178].

102. Orbea CP, Dupuy-McCaulry KL, Morgentahler T. Prevalence and sources of errors in positive airway pressure therapy provisioning. J Clin Sleep Med 2019;15(5):697–704.

103. Mehrtash M, Bakker JP, Ayas N. Predictors of continuous positive airway pressure adherence in patients with obstructive sleep apnea. Lung 2019; 197:115–21.

104. Sawyer AM, Gooneratne NS, Marcus CL, et al. A systematic review of CPAP adherence across age groups: clinical and empiric insights for developing CPAP adherence interventions. Sleep Med Rev 2011;15:343–56.

105. Rowland S, Aiyappan V, Hennessy C, et al. Comparing the efficacy, mask leak, patient adherence, and patient preference of three different CPAP interfaces to treat moderate-severe obstructive sleep apnea. J Clin Sleep Med 2018;14(1):101–8.

106. Shapiro GK, Shapiro CM. Sleep breath. Factors that influence CPAP adherence. Sleep Breath 2010;14(4):323–35.

107. Mastromatto N, Killough N, Keenan BT, et al. CPAP adherence varies with type of patient insurance. Sleep 2018;41(1):402–3.

108. Kuna ST, Shuttleworth D, Chi L, et al. Web-based access to positive airway pressure usage with or without an initial financial incentive improves treatment use in patients with obstructive sleep apnea. Sleep 2015;38(8):1229–36.

109. Malhotra A, Crocker ME, Willes L, et al. Patient engagement using new technology to improve adherence to positive airway pressure therapy: a retrospective analysis. Chest 2018;153:843–50.

110. Lynch S, Blasé A, Erikli L, et al. Retrospective descriptive study of CPAP adherence associated with use of the ResMed myAir application. In: ResMed. 2015. Available at: https://pdfs.semanticscholar.org/bc8e/2341489e89cf76eeae0e76aaccb82a091c92.pdf. Accessed November 14, 2019.

111. Shaughnessy GF, Morgenthaler TI. The effect of patient-facing applications on positive airway pressure therapy adherence: a systematic review. J Clin Sleep Med 2019;15(5):769–77.

112. Isetta V, Leon C, Torres M, et al. Telemedicine-based approach for obstructive sleep apnea management: building evidence. Interact J Med Res 2014;3(1):e6.

113. Guralnick AS, Balachandran JS, Szutenbach S, et al. Educational video to improve CPAP use in patients with obstructive sleep apnoea at risk for poor adherence: a randomised controlled trial. Thorax 2017;72(12):1132–9.

114. Stepnowsky CJ, Palau JJ, Marler MR, et al. Pilot randomized trial of the effect of wireless tele-monitoring on compliance and treatment efficacy in obstructive sleep apnea. J Med Internet Res 2007;9(2):e14. Available at: http://www.jmir.org/2007/2/e14/.

115. Sedkaoui K, et al. Efficiency of a phone coaching program on adherence to continuous positive airway pressure in sleep apnea hypopnea syndrome: a randomized trial. BMC Pulm Med 2015;15:102.

116. Nilius G, Schroeder M, Domanski U, et al. Telemedicine improves continuous positive airway pressure adherence in stroke patients with obstructive sleep apnea in a randomized trial. Respiration 2019;98:410–20.

117. Kotzian ST, Saletu MT, Schwarzinger A, et al. Proactive telemedicine monitoring of sleep apnea treatment improves adherence in people with stroke- a randomized controlled trial (HOPES study). Sleep Med 2019;64:48–55.

118. Tung P, Levitzky YS, Wang R, et al. Obstructive and central sleep apnea and the risk of incident atrial fibrillation in a community cohort of men and women. J Am Heart Assoc 2017;6:e004500.

119. Mendelson M, Vivodtzev I, Tamisier R, et al. CPAP treatment supported by telemedicine does not improve blood pressure in high cardiovascular risk OSA patients: a randomized, controlled trial. Sleep 2014;37:1863–70.

120. Persaud N, Bedard M, Boozary AS, et al. Effect on treatment adherence of distributing essential medicines at no charge: the CLEAN meds randomized clinical trial. JAMA Intern Med 2020;180(1):27–34.

121. Crotti N. ResMed and Philips Respironics use new tools to boost sleep apnea mask adherence. MedCity News; 2016. Available at: https://medcitynews.com/2016/10/resmed/. Accessed January 26, 2020.

122. Woehrle H, Arzt M, Graml A, et al. Effect of a patient engagement tool on positive airway pressure adherence: analysis of a German healthcare provider database. Sleep Med 2018;41:20–6.

123. Isetta V, Navajas D, Montserrat JM, et al. Comparative assessment of several automatic CPAP devices' responses: a bench test study. ERJ Open Res 2015;1(1). 00031-2015.

124. Farré R, Navajas D, Montserrat JM. Technology for noninvasive mechanical ventilation: looking into the black box. ERJ Open Res 2016;2(1). 00004-2016.

125. Koivumaki V, Maasilta P, Bachour A. Oximetry monitoring recommended during PAP initiation for sleep apnea in patients with obesity or nocturnal hypoxemia. J Clin Sleep Med 2018;14(11):1859–63.

126. Stepnowsky C, Zamora T, Barker R, et al. Accuracy of positive airway pressure device-measured apneas and hypopneas: role in treatment followup. Sleep Disord 2013;2013:314589.

127. Rotty MC, Mallet JP, Suehs CM, et al. Is the 2013 American Thoracic Society CPAP-tracking system algorithm useful for managing non-adherence in long-term CPAP-treated patients? Respir Res 2019;20(1):209.

128. Tan M, Keenan B, Staley B, et al. Using an Electronic Health Record (EHR) to identify chronic CPAP users with abnormal HL7 CPAP data. Sleep 2018;41(1):402.

129. Omobomi O, Quan SF. Positional therapy in the management of positional obstructive sleep apnea-a review of the current literature. Sleep Breath 2018;22:297–304. Available at: https://doi-org.proxy.library.upenn.edu/10.1007/s11325-017-1561-y.

130. Ravesloot MJ, White D, Heinzer R, et al. Efficacy of the new generation of devices for positional therapy for patients with positional obstructive sleep apnea: a systematic review of the literature and meta-analysis. J Clin Sleep Med 2017;13(6):813–24.

131. Bignold JJ, Mercer JD, Antic NA, et al. Accurate position monitoring and improved supine-dependent obstructive sleep apnea with a new position recording and supine avoidance device. J Clin Sleep Med 2011;7(4):376–83.

132. Philips sleep position therapy: NightBalance. Available at: https://www.usa.philips.com/c-e/hs/sleep-solutions/nightbalance.html. Accessed January 26, 2020.

133. Advanced Brain monitoring: NightShift. Available at: https://www.advancedbrainmonitoring.com/night-shift/. Accessed January 26, 2020.

134. Berry RB, Uhles ML, Abaluck BK, et al. NightBalance sleep position treatment device versus auto-adjusting positive airway pressure for treatment of positional obstructive sleep apnea. J Clin Sleep Med 2019;15(7):947–56.

135. Levendowski DJ, Seagraves S, Popovic D, et al. Assessment of a neck-based treatment and monitoring device for positional obstructive sleep apnea. J Clin Sleep Med 2014;10(8):863–71.

136. De Ruiter M, Benoist L, de Vries N, et al. Durability of treatment effects of sleep position trainer versus oral appliance therapy in positional OSA: 12-month follow-up of a randomized controlled trial. Sleep Breath 2018;22:441–50.

137. Benoist L, de Ruiter M, de Lange J, et al. A randomized, controlled trial of positional therapy versus oral appliance therapy for position-dependent sleep apnea. Sleep Med 2017;34:109–17.

138. Sutherland K, Cistulli P. Oral appliance therapy for obstructive sleep apnoea: state of the art. J Clin Med 2019;8:2121.

139. Gjerde K, Lehmann S, Naterstad IF, et al. Reliability of an adherence monitoring sensor embedded in an oral appliance used for treatment of obstructive sleep apnoea. J Oral Rehabil 2018;45(2):110–5.

140. Dieltjens M, Vanderveken OM. Oral appliances in obstructive sleep apnea. Healthcare (Basel) 2019;7(4) [pii:E141].

141. SomnoDent with compliance recorder. Available at: https://somnomed.com/en/physicians/compliance-recording/. Accessed January 26, 2020.

142. Sato K, Nakajima T. Review of systematic reviews on mandibular advancement oral appliance for obstructive sleep apnea: the importance of long-term follow-up. Jpn Dent Sci Rev 2020;56(1):32–7.

143. American Academy of Dental Sleep Medicine: oral appliance therapy. Available at: https://aadsm.org/oral_appliance_therapy.php. Accessed January 20, 2020.

144. Inspire sleep apnea innovation: table of contents. Available at: https://professionals.inspiresleep.com/bibliography/. Accessed January 20, 2020.

145. Thaler E, Schwab R, Maurer J, et al. Results of ADHERE upper airway stimulation and predictors of therapy efficacy. Laryngoscope 2019. https://doi.org/10.1002/lary.28286.

146. Dedhia RC, Woodson BT. Standardized reporting for hypoglossal nerve stimulation outcomes. J Clin Sleep Med 2018;14(11):1835–6.

147. Vandervekem OM, Beyers J, Op de Beek S, et al. Development of a clinical pathway and technical aspects of upper airway stimulation therapy for obstructive sleep apnea. Front Neurosci 2017;11:523.

148. Pietzsch JB, Richter AK, Randerath W, et al. Clinical and economic benefits of upper airway stimulation for obstructive sleep apnea in a european setting. Respiration 2019;98:38–47.

149. Woodson BT, Strohl KP, Soose RJ, et al. Upper airway stimulation for obstructive sleep apnea: 5-year outcome. Otolaryngol Head Neck Surg 2018;159(1):194–202.

150. Husser D, Christoph Geller J, Taborsky M, et al. Remote monitoring and clinical outcomes: details on information flow and workflow in the IN-TIME study. Eur Heart J Qual Care Clin Outcomes 2019;5(2):136–44.

151. Parahuleva MS, Soydan N, Divchev D, et al. Home monitoring after ambulatory implanted primary cardiac implantable electronic devices: the home ambulance pilot study. Clin Cardiol 2017;40(11):1068–75.

152. Burri H, Senouf D. Remote monitoring and follow-up of pacemakers and implantable cardioverter defibrillators. Europace 2009;11(6):701–9 [published correction appears in Europace. 2009 Nov;11(11):1569].

153. Chinitz L. Leadless pacemaker for patients with atrioventricular block nets FDA approval. 2020. Available at: https://www.healio.com/cardiology/arrhythmia-disorders/news/online/%7Baf7e44bf-d1b2-4f10-8ffe-5fdad7e3927b%7D/leadless-pacemaker-for-patients-with-atrioventricular-block-nets-fda-approval. Accessed January 26, 2020.

154. American Academy of sleep medicine clinical resources for clinical guidelines and guidelines in development. Available at: https://aasm.org/clinical-resources/practice-standards/practice-guidelines/. Accessed January 26, 2020.

155. Fitzpatrick AL, Wischenka D, Appelhans BM, et al. An evidence-based guide for obesity treatment in primary care. Am J Med 2016;129:115.e1-7.

156. de Vries GE, Hoekema A, Claessen JQPJ, et al. Long-term objective adherence to mandibular advancement device therapy versus continuous positive airway pressure in patients with moderate

obstructive sleep apnea. J Clin Sleep Med 2019; 15(11):1655–63.

157. de Vries GE, Wijkstra PJ, Houwerzijl EJ, et al. Cardiovascular effects of oral appliance therapy in obstructive sleep apnea: a systematic review and meta-analysis. Sleep Med Rev 2018;40: 55–68.

158. Cillo JE, Robertson N, Dattilo DJ. Maxillomandibular advancement for obstructive sleep apnea is associated with very long-term overall sleep-related quality-of-life improvement. J Oral Maxillofac Surg 2020;78:109–17.

159. Benca RM, Teodorescu M. Sleep physiology and disorders in aging and dementia. Handb Clin Neurol 2019;167:477–93.

160. Zolfaghari S, Yao C, Thompson C, et al. Effects of menopause on sleep quality and sleep disorders: Canadian Longitudinal Study on Aging. Menopause 2020;27(3):295–304.

161. Cowan DC, Livingston E. Obstructive sleep apnoea syndrome and weight loss: review. Sleep Disord 2012;163296:11.

162. Friberg D, Carlsson-Nordlander B, Larsson H, et al. UPPP for habitual snoring: a 5-year follow-up with respiratory sleep recordings. Laryngoscope 1995; 105(5 Pt 1):519–22.

163. Boot H, van Wegen R, Poublon RM, et al. Long-term results of uvulopalatopharyngoplasty for obstructive sleep apnea syndrome. Laryngoscope 2000;110(3 Pt 1):469–75.

164. Levin BC, Becker GD. Uvulopalatopharyngoplasty for snoring: long-term results. Laryngoscope 1994;104(9):1150–2.

165. Neagoe R, Muresan M, Timofte D, et al. Long-term outcomes of laparoscopic sleeve gastrectomy - a single-center prospective observational study. Wideochir Inne Tech Maloinwazyjne 2019;14(2):242–8.

166. Wang SH, Keenan BT, Wiemken A, et al. Effect of weight loss on upper airway anatomy and the apnea hypopnea index: the importance of tongue fat. Am J Respir Crit Care Med 2020. https://doi.org/10.1164/rccm.201903-0692OC.

167. Callahan ZM, Su B, Kuchta K, et al. Five-year results of endoscopic gastrojejunostomy revision (transoral outlet reduction) for weight gain after gastric bypass. Surg Endosc 2019. https://doi.org/10.1007/s00464-019-07003-6.

168. Farré R, Navajas D, Montserrat JM. Is telemedicine a key tool for improving continuous positive airway pressure adherence in patients with sleep apnea? Am J Respir Crit Care Med 2018;197:12–4.

169. CVS HealthHub: a new approach to healthcare. Available at: https://www.cvs.com/content/healthhub/sleep-apnea. Accessed June 17, 2020.

170. Walgreens: a new way to find care. Available at: https://www.walgreens.com/findcare/services. Accessed January 26, 2020.

171. Definitive healthcare: the top 3 most important pharmacy mergers and acquisitions of 2018. 2019. Available at: https://blog.definitivehc.com/top-3-pharmacy-acquisitions-2018. Accessed January 26, 2020.

172. Luo J, Wu M, Gopukumar D, et al. Big data application in biomedical research and health care: a literature review. Biomed Inform Insights 2016;8:1–10.

173. Price WN, Gerke S, Cohen IG. Potential liability for physicians using artificial intelligence. JAMA 2019; 322(18):1765–6.

174. Hwang TJ, Kesselheim AS, Vokinger KN. Lifecycle regulation of artificial intelligence– and machine learning–based software devices in medicine. JAMA 2019;322(23):2285–6.

175. Shi H, Zhao H, Liu Y, et al. Systematic analysis of a military wearable device based on a multi-level fusion framework: research directions. Sensors 2019;19(12):2651.

176. Kamišalić A, Fister I, Turkanović M, et al. Sensors and functionalities of non-invasive wrist-wearable devices: a review. Sensors 2018;18(6):1714.

177. Walch O, Huang Y, Forger D, et al. Sleep stage prediction with raw acceleration and photoplethysmography heart rate data derived from a consumer wearable device. Sleep 2019;20(20): 1–19.

178. Auerbach AD. Evaluating digital health tools—prospective, experimental, and real world. JAMA Intern Med 2019;179(6):840–1.

179. Chen CE, Harrington RA, Desai SA, et al. Characteristics of digital health studies registered in ClinicalTrials.gov. JAMA Intern Med 2019;179(6): 838–40.

180. Guk K, Han G, Lim J, et al. Evolution of wearable devices with real-time disease monitoring for personalized healthcare. Nanomaterials 2019; 9(6):813.

181. Qureshi F, Krishnan S. Wearable hardware design for the internet of medical things (IoMT). Sensors 2018;18(11):3812.

182. Ko PR, Kientz JA, Choe EK, et al. Consumer sleep technologies: a review of the landscape. J Clin Sleep Med 2015;11(12):1455–61.

183. Khosla S, Deak MC, Gault D, et al. Consumer sleep technologies: how to balance the promises of new technology with evidence-based medicine and clinical guidelines. J Clin Sleep Med 2019;15(1): 163–5.

184. Sharman JE, O'Brien E, Alpert B, et al. Lancet commission on hypertension group position statement on the global improvement of accuracy standards for devices that measure blood pressure. J Hypertens 2019. https://doi.org/10.1097/HJH.0000000000002246.

185. US Food and Drug Administration. Digital health software precertification (Pre-Cert) program.

Available at: https://www.fda.gov/MedicalDevices/DigitalHealth/DigitalHealthPreCertProgram/default.htm. Accessed November 14, 2019.

186. Apple healthcare. 2020. Available at: https://www.apple.com/healthcare/. Accessed January 26, 2020.

187. Gramling, A. How Hospitals are using Apple HealthKit and ResearchKit. In 2020 Healthcare IT Leaders. 2015. Available at: https://www.healthcareitleaders.com/blog/how-hospitals-are-using-apples-healthkit-and-researchkit/. Accessed January 26, 2020.

188. Oschner Health System. Hypertension digital medicine program. Available at: https://www.ochsner.org/hypertension-digital-medicine. Accessed January 26, 2020.

189. Cohen IG, Mello MM. Big data, big tech, and protecting patient privacy. JAMA 2019;322(12):1141–2.

190. National Sleep Research Resources (funded by the National Heart, Lung, and Blood Institute). Available at: https://sleepdata.org/. Accessed January 26, 2020.

EHR Integration of PAP Devices in Sleep Medicine Implementation in the Clinical Setting

Tereza Cervenka, MD, Conrad Iber, MD*

KEYWORDS

- Electronic health record (EHR) • CPAP adherence • Noninvasive ventilator (NIV) • Telemedicine
- Interoperability • Machine learning • Data warehouse

KEY POINTS

- Positive airway pressure therapy integration is a component of electronic health record (EHR) sleep medicine optimization.
- EHR optimization facilitates telehealth in continuous care population health.
- A coordinated care plan can leverage early telehealth interventions.

BACKGROUND

The growth of electronic health record (EHR) use has reached 67% to 96%[1] across the United States, based on state reporting of certification to meaningful use, and surveys show a narrow field of 4 vendors providing EHRs for 69%[2] of hospital facilities. Barriers to EHR use have included cost, variations in EHR implementations, and some unintended consequences. Conincident with rapid growth, improvements in process, efficiency and error reduction have also been verified The adoption of the additional components within the EHR, including interoperability, telemedicine, patient portals, database housing, trigger alerts, and increasing device integration, have provided a fertile setting for housing most activities in sleep medicine in the EHR. Recent interoperability in some EHRs likely mitigates process delays and errors of omission created by unavailable health information in external systems of care. EHR-centered database housing with predictive analytics and timely intervention provide the best opportunities for improving population health in a chronic disease setting of common sleep disorders.

The recent pandemic has been a forcing function requiring rapid rollout of telemedicine and promoting interest in device integration both within a single EHR sign-in. In the context of diverse systems storing patient information across the United States, this visit model encourages leveraging all aspects of data gathering, including automated population of EHRs from devices as well rapid interoperability for incorporating patient health information from care in other systems. The autointegration single EHR sign-in can be provided through direct EHR interface and processing or assisted by a middleware solution incorporated in the EHR. When deployed more fully, assistance from predictive analytics could be triggered at the time the EHR is opened for case management at diagnosis, therapy initiation, or touchpoints in long-term monitoring could be added to optimize timely care and resource allocation in the chronic obstructive sleep apnea. This discussion provides perspective on the opportunity for direct EHR integration process for positive airway pressure (PAP)

Department of Medicine, Pulmonary, Allergy, Critical Care and Sleep Medicine, M Health Fairview and University of Minnesota, 420 Delaware Street Southeast, Minneapolis, MN 55455, USA
* Corresponding author.
E-mail address: iberx001@umn.edu

Sleep Med Clin 15 (2020) 377–382
https://doi.org/10.1016/j.jsmc.2020.06.001
1556-407X/20/© 2020 Elsevier Inc. All rights reserved.

(and eventually noninvasive ventilator [NIV] devices) with presentation of data and clinical examples from an existing data set.

COMPONENTS OF ELECTRONIC HEALTH RECORD OPTIMIZATION FOR SLEEP MEDICINE PRACTICE

Optimization of EHR for sleep medicine requires more than computational processes. The presentation to providers should provide ready access to information in a familiar format with helpful structures to facilitate best practices. The landing page for EHR for medical specialties typically is highly customized with the specialty format, with rapid button or tabular access displaying landing fields for discrete data that are familiar and needed. In sleep medicine, this often includes sleep diagnostic results, sleep scales, PAP information, durable medical equipment (DME) comments, and insomnia care strategies (see example of tabular format in **Fig. 1**), with sleep medicine discrete data field information pulled automatically into templates similar to standard

		5/8/20 0000		5/9/20 0000		5/10/20 0000
PAP Device						
PAP Therapy Discontinued						
How old is your current device?						
Where did you obtain your current PAP device if applicable?						
PAP setup date (if new set up or replacement)						
Where do you get your device and supplies?						
Mask						
Which type of mask?						
Mask Size						
How old is your current mask?						
Device and Settings						
Vendor						
Daily Event						
EPAP Min Auto CPAP/ASV		10.0		10.0		10.0
EPAP Max Auto CPAP/ASV		20.0		20.0		20.0
(EPR) Expiratory Pressure Reliefe type		FULLTIME		FULLTIME		FULLTIME
(EPR) Expiratory Pressure Relief level		TWO		TWO		TWO
Total Mask Events		4		2		4
Target IPAP (95% of Target)		11.4		12		12.36
Hypopnea Index - Daily		0.5		0.6		1.7
Apnea Index - Daily		0.5		2.4		0.4
Obstructive Apnea Index - Daily		0.2		1.3		0.4
Central Apnea Index - Daily		0.2		0.5		0
Unknown Apnea Index - Daily		0		0.5		0
Rolling Averages						
95% of leak in litres per second i		0.46		0.72		0.7
95% of leak in LPM		27.6		43.2		42
95% OF Leak in litres Rolling Average 14 D		28.96		30.24		31.44
95% OF Leak in litres Rolling Average 30 D		28.61		29.57		29.88
95% OF Leak in litres Rolling Average 180 D		30.22		30.35		30.46
Number days on		99		100		101
AHI - Daily		1.0		3.0		2.2
AHI Rolling Average 14 D		2.85		2.75		2.59
AHI Rolling Average 30 D		3.36		3.32		3.22
AHI Rolling Average 180 D		3.15		3.15		3.14
Target IPAP (95% of Target) 14 d average		11.5		11.6		11.6
Target IPAP (95% of Target) 30 d average		11.7		11.7		11.7
% compliance greater than four hours rolling average 14 d		100		100		100
% compliance greater than four hours rolling average 30 d		100		100		100
% compliance greater than four hours rolling average 180 d		98		99		99
Time mask on face 14 d average		467		473		465
Hours mask on face 14 d average		7.8		7.9		7.8
Time mask on face 30 d average		484		483		483
Compliance Greater than 4 H		Yes		Yes		Yes
COMPLIANCE (TOTAL TIME MASK ON FACE) - Daily		473		450		373

Tabs: Sleep History Questio... | Diagnostic Results | Sleep Scales | MA History | PAP Therapy WorkSheet | SLP Comprehensive DME | Insomnia Care

Search (Alt+Comma) — Hide All Show All

Sidebar: PAP Device ✓ | Mask ✓ | Device and Settings ✓ | Daily Event ✓ | Rolling Averages ✓ | Rolling Averages ✓ | PAP Therapy Comfortable Co... ✓

Expanded | View All — 1m 5m 10m 15m 30m 1h 2h 4h

Fig. 1. Example of sleep medicine EHR landing page for customized visit with topical tabs for each discrete data field. ASV, adpative servo ventilation; EPAP, expiratory positive airway pressure; IPAP, inspiratory positive airway pressure.

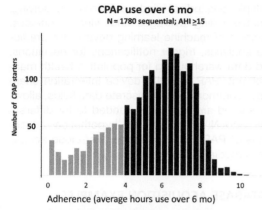

Fig. 2. Distribution of CPAP use in hours averaged over 6 months; early use at 30 days to 60 days has positive predictive value of 70% to 80% for 6-month use of less than 4 hours; the early poor users (in *gray*) are escalated to 2 weeks coaching.

self-populating areas of the visit. Interoperability allows search of the entire chart for sleep medicine testing and notes from outside the system of care and typically is deployed within regional EHR sharing areas.

Additional tools include an array of templates, including provider templates with fields prepopulated from extracted data fields (examples include continuous PAP [CPAP] compliance data, sleep scales, and metrics), templates for interchart communication by staff, templates for letters, and chart portal patient messaging (examples include driving limitations and cognitive behavioral coaching). Telemedicine can be initiated through the same specialty chart site and asynchronous communications from and to patients, including attached questionnaires or scanned materials to facilitate the visit. Preformed order formats and internal archived communications, for instance, a coordinated care or DME provider note, can be standardized to reduce practice variations and to prevent errors. Communications can be optimized by assigning pools to manage communications in a cross-cover fashion and by scheduling reminders for completing tasks. More detailed recommendations for EHR optimization and choices for metrics can be obtained through the American Academy of Sleep Medicine.[3]

DEVICE INTEGRATION
Durable Medical Equipment Structures

Asynchronous and often inconveniently timed and directed PAP data information provided by facsimile has been widely replaced by cloud-based solutions. These may be sufficient for single-practitioner settings and for self-monitoring by patients but more challenging for large distributed health care systems employing

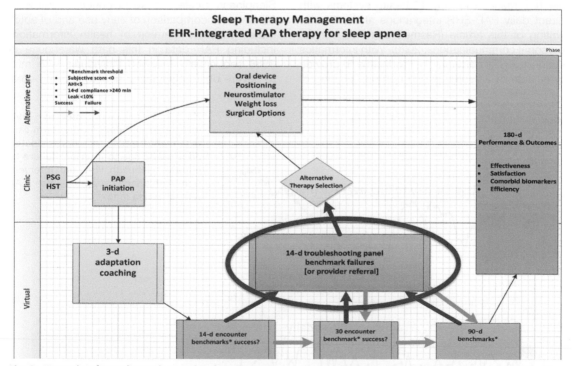

Fig. 3. Example of coordinated care plan for management of poor CPAP use by benchmark and intervention by a team trained in management strategies and motivational interviewing. HST, home sleep test; PSG, polysomnography.

varying practice patterns and with fewer cloud access sites spread across larger geographic areas, particularly if primary care plays a larger part in chronic disease management in common sleep disorders. Standardization and supervised DME practices and daily autointegration into the EHR with incorporation of predictive analytics, trigger alerts, and coordinated telemedicine care serve larger populations across multiple contact sites. The role of predictive analytics and machine learning shows promise in sleep medicine. Although through cloud-based software multiple DME vendors can be integrated into an EHR, it may be preferable in the setting of variable DME practices to have a limited number or a single DME with standardized practices to facilitate setup, modem initialization, and integration for EHR documentation of home interventions and communications.

Electronic Health Record Device Integration

Device manufacturers offer capability of EHR interface support for all certified EHRs although the cost and development of modifying destination EHR structures are substantial. The first EHR-PAP integration requested by a health care system to 2 vendors occurred in 2014 to 2015.[4] This process requires an initial build on the destination EHR side with internal informatics support or adopting a middleware solution. The internal software barrier has resulted in only 17 health systems with direct daily PAP-EHR integrations at the time of writing of this article (Resmed and Respironics, personal communications, 2020). With informatics support, EHRs certainly are modifiable to provide daily data of all settings and outputs, plotting of multiple longitudinal windows for problem solving, variable rolling averages and window choices, insertion of machine learning devices for predictive analytics, trigger notifications for deviations, and data warehousing for population health management. PAP and NIV device integration share some common sites for discrete data fields, allowing shared areas to be expanded to for different PAP and NIV devices. The hypothetical advantages of PAP-EHR integration over cloud access are immediate within visit access.

DATABASE ACQUISITION EXAMPLES

Data warehouses can be queried or automated to meet provide indicators for care on individual patients and can be used in quality reporting and continuous improvement projects. Integrated PAP data in obstructive sleep apnea has an initial start date providing a history from which abandonment may be detected more easily and can be used to predict long-term use. In 1 longitudinal study of CPAP adherence, 1530 patients starting CPAP for AHI>/=15 with telehealth interventions based on trigger thresholds showed low abandonment rates of 2% to 6% over 6 months. Six-month CPAP adherence was predicted by early CPAP use,[5] with less than 5% of variance attributable to other measures, including age, gender, apnea-hypopnea index (AHI), body mass index, Epworth Sleepiness Scale, or socioeconomic status.[5,6] Subsequent comparison of early use and of automated machine learning of health information, including PAP data in this data warehouse in 3588 sequentially followed individuals with mild to severe obstructive sleep apnea, showed early

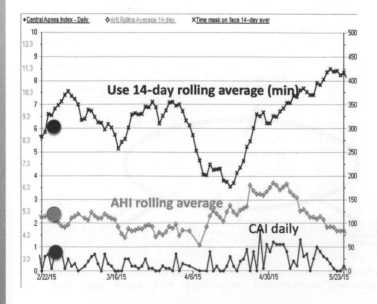

Fig. 4. Example of use of EHR-integrated PAP data in long-term care for identification of unanticipated poor usage due to interface failure to initiate telehealth visit and intervention. AHI, apnea hypopnea index; CAI, central apnea index.

CPAP use and machine learning at 13 days to 30 days had high positive predictive value for CPAP use at 6 months.[7] These strategies to leverage data to improve access and processes are vital to identifying the subgroup of individuals (**Fig. 2**) who are identified early with interventions to improve use or identify alternative therapies. Although it is likely that the addition of machine learning quickly captures additional metrics to improve timely prediction of poor CPAP adherence, interventional trials are necessary to inform effectiveness of interventions.

CLINICAL CARE APPROACHES

Long-term CPAP adherence is an ongoing problem that begs an ongoing management strategy.[8] Though benefits of long-term CPAP use remain controversial[9–13]; there are ample data to support optimizing continuing care with CPAP use.[14–18] A coordinated care plan can leverage early telehealth interventions based on established benchmarks or automated triggers and employ interventions by trained CPAP coaches using standardized management strategies, motivational methods[19–21] and diversion to alternative therapies for those failing CPAP use (**Fig. 3**). Long-term database monitoring identifies unanticipated drops in CPAP use (**Fig. 4**) or abandonment (defined as <20-minute daily use). The integration of automated or queried data triggers based on benchmarks allows interventions in long-term care and weekly panel review of cases with benchmark exceptions by a sleep medicine physician and coaching team. Patients abandoning therapy due to relocation, death, or alternative therapy choice carry a database identifier and can be removed from the CPAP use monitoring panel.

SUMMARY

EHR optimization and data integration can be a provider's companion in optimizing continuing care. When leveraged with exception management and coordinated care coaching intervention, patients have a greater opportunity to access alternative therapy interventions. Sleep medicine likely will see increasing integration of interoperability, device reporting, and artificial intelligence to augment care management strategies in conjunction with targeted rather than timed telehealth interventions.[22]

CONFLICT OF INTERESTS

Both authors are investigators for Inspire Medical and neither has commercial relationships with EHR or PAP device manufacturers.

DISCLOSURE

Fairview Health Systems provided support for this sleep medicine optimization.

REFERENCES

1. Myrick KL, OD, Ogburn DF, et al. (EHR)/electronic medical record (EMR) system and physicians that have a certified EHR/EMR system. In: National Electronic Health Records Survey. 2017. Available at: https://www.cdc.gov/nchs/data/nehrs/2017 _NEHRS _Web _Table _EHR _State.pdf. Accessed July 17, 2020.
2. Roth M. In EMR market share wars, EPIC and cerner triumph yet again. In: HealthLeaders. 2019. Available at: https://www.healthleadersmedia.com/innovation/emr-market-share-wars-epic-and-cerner-triumph-yet-again. Accessed July 17, 2020.
3. Hwang D, Bae C, Iber C, et al. A handbook for optimizing EHR use in sleep medicine. Darien (IL): American Academy of Sleep Medicine; 2017.
4. ResMed and fairview health services introduce integration of sleep and respiratory therapy data into EHR system. PRNewswire 2014.
5. Iber C, Kazaglis L, Steffens H, et al. CPAP adherence in sleep apnea managed with virtual care and EHR integration. Sleep 2017;40:A195.
6. Billings ME, Auckley D, Benca R, et al. Race and residential socioeconomics as predictors of CPAP adherence. Sleep 2011;34(12):1653–8.
7. Araujo M, Kazaglis L, Bhojwani R, et al. Machine learning to predict PAP adherence and compliance in tele-health management. Sleep 2018;41:A400–1.
8. Weaver TE. Don't start celebrating–CPAP adherence remains a problem. J Clin Sleep Med 2013;9(6):551–2.
9. McEvoy RD, Antic NA, Heeley E, et al. CPAP for prevention of cardiovascular events in obstructive sleep apnea. N Engl J Med 2016;375(10):919–31.
10. Mokhlesi B, Ayas NT. Cardiovascular events in obstructive sleep apnea - can CPAP therapy SAVE lives? N Engl J Med 2016;375(10):994–6.
11. Javaheri S, Martinez-Garcia MA, Campos-Rodriguez F. CPAP treatment and cardiovascular prevention: we need to change the design and implementation of our trials. Chest 2019;156(3):431–7.
12. Quan SF, Budhiraja R, Batool-Anwar S, et al. Lack of impact of mild obstructive sleep apnea on sleepiness, mood and quality of life. Southwest J Pulm Crit Care 2014;9(1):44–56.
13. Quan SF, Budhiraja R, Clarke DP, et al. Impact of treatment with continuous positive airway pressure (CPAP) on weight in obstructive sleep apnea. J Clin Sleep Med 2013;9(10):989–93.
14. Richards KC, Gooneratne N, Dicicco B, et al. CPAP adherence may slow 1-year cognitive decline in

older adults with mild cognitive impairment and apnea. J Am Geriatr Soc 2019;67(3):558–64.

15. Pepin JL, Jullian-Desayes I, Sapene M, et al. Multimodal remote monitoring of high cardiovascular risk patients with OSA initiating CPAP: a randomized trial. Chest 2019;155(4):730–9.

16. Schwarz EI, Schlatzer C, Rossi VA, et al. Effect of CPAP withdrawal on BP in OSA: data from three randomized controlled trials. Chest 2016;150(6):1202–10.

17. Weaver TE, Mancini C, Maislin G, et al. Continuous positive airway pressure treatment of sleepy patients with milder obstructive sleep apnea: results of the CPAP Apnea Trial North American Program (CATNAP) randomized clinical trial. Am J Respir Crit Care Med 2012;186(7):677–83.

18. Gottlieb DJ, Punjabi NM, Mehra R, et al. CPAP versus oxygen in obstructive sleep apnea. N Engl J Med 2014;370(24):2276–85.

19. Lai AYK, Fong DYT, Lam JCM, et al. The efficacy of a brief motivational enhancement education program on CPAP adherence in OSA: a randomized controlled trial. Chest 2014;146(3):600–10.

20. Bakker JP, Weaver TE, Parthasarathy S, et al. Adherence to CPAP: what should we be aiming for, and how can we get there? Chest 2019;155(6):1272–87.

21. Deng T, Wang Y, Sun M, et al. Stage-matched intervention for adherence to CPAP in patients with obstructive sleep apnea: a randomized controlled trial. Sleep Breath 2013;17(2):791–801.

22. Pepin JL, Tamisier R, Hwang D, et al. Does remote monitoring change OSA management and CPAP adherence? Respirology 2017;22(8):1508–17.

Telemedicine and the Management of Insomnia

Caleb Hsieh, MD, MS, Talayeh Rezayat, DO, MPH, Michelle R. Zeidler, MD, MS*

KEYWORDS

• Insomnia • Telemedicine • Cognitive behavior therapy for insomnia (CBT-i)

KEY POINTS

• Insomnia is a highly prevalent disorder with significant medical and economic consequences best treated with cognitive behavioral therapy for insomnia (CBT-i).
• Behavioral therapies administered through telemedicine are well validated and effective including tele-CBT-i.
• Tele-CBT-i can be delivered through fully directed care with a behavioral therapist or through a self-directed Web or mobile app with varying degrees of therapist interaction.
• Multiple randomized studies as well as meta-analyses show efficacy of both fully directed and self-directed tele-CBT-i.
• Tele-CBT-i increases access for patients with insomnia that are geographically remote.

INTRODUCTION

Insomnia is highly prevalent in the general population with significant economic and social ramifications. Although the exact prevalence of insomnia in the United States is unknown, approximately 30% to 40% of US adults will report insomnia symptoms at some point over a year and approximately 10% will meet criteria for a diagnosis of chronic insomnia. Prevalence of insomnia is increasing, with certain populations, including women and veterans, being more susceptible to developing insomnia.[1] The economic burden due to insomnia is high and includes missed work days and increased rates of occupational and motor vehicle accidents.[2,3] In addition, insomnia is linked to the development of comorbid mental health and medical conditions, including depression, hypertension, diabetes, and heart disease, among others.[3,4]

Treatment options for insomnia include pharmacologic and nonpharmacologic pathways with multiple clinical guidelines recommending utilization of nonpharmacologic approaches, specifically cognitive behavioral therapy (CBT-i), for first-line treatment of insomnia.[5,6] Although CBT-i is clearly effective and durable for the treatment of insomnia, there are inadequate CBT-i providers to treat the large and rapidly growing insomnia patient population. In addition, most insomnia providers reside within metropolitan areas, which further exacerbates shortages in rural areas. There are currently only 300 CBT-i providers certified by the Society of Behavioral Sleep medicine within the United States.[6] Within the US Department of Veterans Affairs, there were 112 full-time mental health physician and psychologist providers nationwide in 2012 for a population of veterans with diagnosed insomnia estimated to reach a half-million by 2020.[7] Many of these veterans as well as nonveteran patients live in rural areas where the closest provider is often multiple hours away and may be geographically inaccessible during periods of the year.[2] Shortages of CBT-i providers translates to longer appointment wait times, shorter patient visits to accommodate higher volume, and clinician burnout, as well as a need for the primary physician to treat patients with insomnia with pharmacologic therapies rather than referring for CBT-i.

Pulmonary, Critical Care and Sleep Medicine, David Geffen School of Medicine at UCLA, 10833 Le Conte Avenue, 43-229 CHS, Los Angeles, CA, USA
* Corresponding author.
E-mail address: MZeidler@mednet.ucla.edu

Sleep Med Clin 15 (2020) 383–390
https://doi.org/10.1016/j.jsmc.2020.05.004
1556-407X/20/Published by Elsevier Inc.

sleep.theclinics.com

Given the rapid technological advances of recent years, there has been a proliferation of options for the management and treatment of insomnia. Tele-CBT-i, either with a provider or through self-directed CBT-i via the Web or mobile applications, has generated excitement as a bridge to address the barriers to care for a large population of patients.[8] This article reviews and evaluates the evidence for the various telemedicine modalities for the treatment of insomnia.

DEFINITIONS
Insomnia

The International Classification of Sleep Disorders defines insomnia as difficulty with sleep onset, maintenance, duration, or quality, with resulting daytime symptoms in the setting of adequate opportunity and environment for sleep.[9] Insomnia is further categorized as short-term insomnia lasting less than 3 months or chronic insomnia, persisting longer than 3 months.

Cognitive and Behavioral Treatment for Insomnia

Cognitive behavioral therapy for insomnia is considered first-line treatment for insomnia, and has been shown to be more effective and durable than pharmacologic therapy with fewer side effects.[10] Skills and techniques such as stimulus control (behavioral instructions to enhance the bed as stimulus for sleep), sleep restriction (reducing the time in bed to align with sleep time), relaxation, and developing healthy sleep habits help patients address various predisposing, precipitating, and perpetuating causes of chronic insomnia. CBT-i is traditionally completed through face-to-face office visits over a course of 6 to 8 weeks with weekly or every-other-week visits.[7]

Given the time and resource intensity required for CBT-i, brief behavioral therapy for insomnia (BBT-i) was developed as an abridged form of CBT-i accessible to a wider range of clinicians.[11] BBT-i has demonstrated efficacy[12,13] and can reach a larger pool of patients through the training of nonsleep mental health providers to deliver therapy. BBT-i was originally derived from CBT-i and is completed over a shorter duration of 4 weeks (4 sessions) and focuses on sleep restriction and stimulus control[12] (**Fig. 1**). BBT-i is traditionally done with 2 in-person visits and 2 telephone visits and represents a hybrid of in-office and telemedicine services. Those patients who continue to have residual symptoms following BBT-i can be referred for CBT-i to address components not covered in BBT-i.

Telemedicine

The American Academy of Sleep Medicine separates sleep telemedicine into 2 types: synchronous and asynchronous.[2] In synchronous interactions, patients and providers are separated by distance, but interact in real time via bi-directional telecommunication.[2] The patient may be at a sleep laboratory, a designated clinic, or at their home (provided adequate technical specifications are met) while the provider similarly works from any location with a secure networking connection. Besides the technological intermediary interface, there may be little to distinguish the interaction from an in-person office clinic visit. In asynchronous interactions, patients and providers are separated by both distance and time using "store and forward" technology. Home sleep apnea testing and interpretations, as well as secure e-messaging, are examples already commonly in use. Self-directed care mechanisms are another rapidly growing subset of telemedicine that include mobile phone applications (apps) and Web-based programs that can be enhanced by the use of smart devices or wearable devices. These modalities can be fully self-directed without provider interaction or partially directed, usually through asynchronous interactions. For example, a patient could use a CBT-i app to transmit data on sleep onset and fragmentation through both a sleep diary and from an actigraphy-enabled smart watch. A provider then receives the data and provides counseling on sleep restriction.

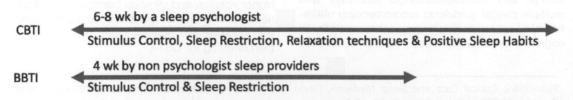

Fig. 1. CBT-i compared with BBT-i. CBT-i is the gold standard treatment for insomnia. It is provided by a sleep-trained psychologist over 6 to 8 sessions and uses stimulus control, sleep restriction, relaxation techniques, and positive sleep habits. BBT-i can be provided by a trained nonpsychologist. BBT-i is shorter in duration (4 sessions) and uses stimulus control and sleep restriction.

TELEMEDICINE FOR INSOMNIA

Although telemedicine has traditionally implied the exchange of health-related services between the clinician and patient via telecommunications, expanding technology enables telemedicine for insomnia to use both synchronous and asynchronous modalities, as well as self-directed care mechanisms using varying levels of clinician support (**Fig. 2**). With synchronous telemedicine, patients with insomnia in varied geographic locations work directly with a CBT-i provider, either in a one-on-one or group setting. Asynchronous telemedicine modalities allow patients to use self-directed insomnia treatments through Web or mobile apps, some of which have access to a provider for support and clarifications.

Telemedicine has significant potential to expand access to nonpharmacologic treatment of insomnia, although with pros and cons depending on the modality used. On one end of the spectrum, completely self-directed therapy is almost universally accessible with relatively low costs compared with using a CBT-i therapist. This may result in a therapy that may be too general and superficial, especially for patients with more severe insomnia or insomnia with comorbid conditions. Conversely, fully directed therapy allows for greater depth of treatment, but as such is much more time and resource intensive (**Table 1**).

Research studies have investigated the efficacy of both synchronous and asynchronous CBT-i in comparison with either an insomnia therapy waitlist or with face-to-face behavioral therapy for insomnia.

Fully Directed Individual Telehealth Cognitive Behavioral Therapy for Insomnia

In recent decades, telemedicine-based psychotherapy has been shown to be effective in the adjunctive treatment of numerous mental health conditions when compared with face-to-face psychotherapy.[14,15] Within the umbrella of fully directed telemedicine-delivered CBT-i, various options exist with varying degrees of clinician interaction, including videoconferencing, telephone visits, and synchronous text chats. For technical and administrative considerations, the reader is referred to the best practices consensus statement published by the American Telehealth Association and the American Psychiatric Association.[16]

Although there have not been large-scale comparisons of face-to-face CBT-i versus telemedicine-delivered CBT-i, preliminary results of 30 patients from a study using the American Academy of Sleep Medicine video telemedicine platform indicate that telemedicine-delivered CBT-i is noninferior to face-to-face delivery.[17] Gieselmann and Pietrowsky[18] randomized individuals

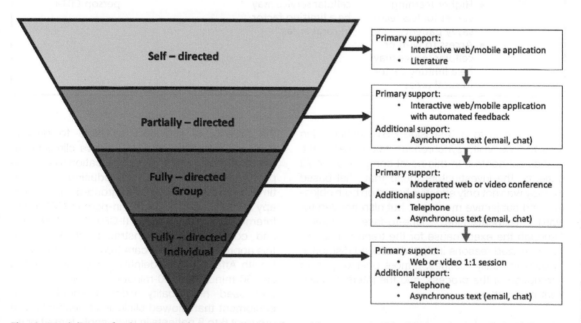

Fig. 2. Modalities of tele-CBT-i with varying levels of provider support. Tele-CBT-i can range from fully self-directed to fully directed with variations in-between. Self-directed CBT-i delivered primarily via the Internet or mobile application is widely available and readily accessible to many patients. Self-directed therapy alone requires few resources but may not be as appropriate for patients with more individualized needs. Varying layers of clinician support can be added to provide better direction for patients from partial to full support.

Table 1
Positive and negative features of tele-CBT-i modalities

Features of tele-CBT-i	Self-Directed Internet/Mobile CBT-i	Partially Directed Internet/Mobile CBT-i	Fully Directed Group Telemedicine CBT-i	Fully Directed Individual Telemedicine CBT-i
Positive	• Least time and resource burden on clinicians • Fewest barriers to accessibility • Allows integration with other wearable devices	• Less time and resource burden on clinicians • Allows for support and feedback that may improve insomnia outcomes • Variable degree of personalization/individualization of treatment depending on site	• Less time and resource burden on clinicians • Allows social support among participants and positive group dynamics	• Most flexibility for treatment individualization/personalization • Most similar to traditional in-person CBT-i
Negative	• Limited personalization/individualization of treatment • Lack of regulation or quality control of Web sites and apps • Increased health-information privacy and security risks • Higher learning curves for less tech-savvy patients • Access to wi-fi or cellular service may be a limiting factor in rural areas	• Lack of regulation or quality control of Web sites and apps • Increased health-information privacy and security risks • Higher learning curves for less tech-savvy patients • Access to wi-fi or cellular service may be a limiting factor in rural areas	• Requires synchronous interactions • Limited by patient social anxieties or negative group dynamics • Less accessible than self-directed therapy	• More time and resource intensive than other tele-modalities • Requires synchronous interactions • Potential adverse effects on the clinician-patient therapeutic relationship as compared with in-person CBT-i

with insomnia to a 3-session BBT-i either using face-to-face visit, synchronous text-based chat, or wait-list control. In this novel comparison of 73 patients, the investigators found that chat-based therapy was not only effective based on both objective and subjective measures, but also trended toward outperforming face-to-face therapy. Although the exact cause for the trend is unclear, hypothesized reasons included reduced disruption to patients' daily routines, a more positive patient perception of the process, and the Internet-based treatment setting.

Fully Directed Group Telehealth Cognitive Behavioral Therapy for Insomnia

Although directed individual tele-CBT-i addresses issues of geographic access, it does not address the paucity of providers available to provide CBT-i. Group-directed CBT-i allows clinicians to deliver therapy, training, and education to multiple patients simultaneously, thus reducing costs and time burdens. The efficacy of group-directed therapy is likely similar to both in-person CBT-i and Internet-delivered CBT-i (I-CBT-i).[19] Gehrman and colleagues[20] demonstrated efficacy using this approach to deliver care through the Veterans Health Affairs in Philadelphia. They implemented six 60-minute to 90-minute session protocols and used high-quality video teleconferencing equipment that allowed clinicians to either view a group of 6 to 8 patients in wide-angle format or individual group members close up. In 214 veterans, there were notable improvements in mean insomnia severity index (ISI) (measure of insomnia from 0 to 28 with higher scores indicating worse insomnia), sleep latency, and sleep efficiency that were comparable to published data on group CBT-i. In the preceding format with a teleconference clinician, tele-CBT-i likely suffers from many of the same barriers faced by traditional face-to-face group sessions (eg, patient concerns about group dynamics, limited accessibility, or negative group dynamics).[21]

Holmqvist and colleagues[22] randomized patients with insomnia to either clinical visit telehealth group CBT-i (the patient physically attends their primary care clinic and then undergoes CBT-i via telehealth with a remote provider) or a Web-based CBT-i completed from their home without therapist contact. Both groups completed identical modules. There were significant and similar improvements in insomnia symptoms in both groups, although there was a preference trend for Web-based treatment.

Self-Directed Internet/App Cognitive Behavioral Therapy for Insomnia

The most readily available option for CBT-i is self-directed "on-line" therapy, otherwise known as "Web-based," "Internet-based," "mobile application," or "Internet-delivered" CBT-i (I-CBT-i). I-CBT-i pairs patients with educational material and varying levels of feedback and support directed through either an automated computer program or an insomnia provider. There are more than a dozen different self-directed I-CBT-i options with proprietary solutions and varying efficacy, although many of these programs lack evidence-based data regarding their product. On the whole, randomized studies of self-directed therapy delivered via Internet or mobile devices have demonstrated efficacy for the treatment of insomnia. Use is limited by access to a wireless network or cellular service as well as access to a compatible device to use the program and at least some degree of computer literacy.

Studies as early as 2004 evaluated the use of I-CBT-i for the treatment of insomnia[23] with subsequent multiple randomized studies and 3 meta-analyses being published since then.[24–26] These studies have evaluated the use of I-CBT-i with face-to-face CBT-i visits, placebo, and I-CBT-i with varying levels of support.

Self-Directed Internet/App Cognitive Behavioral Therapy for Insomnia Versus Face-to-Face Cognitive Behavioral Therapy for Insomnia

Blom and colleagues[19] evaluated 48 patients randomized to I-CBT-i or face-to-face group CBT-i for 8 weeks and 6 months of follow-up. I-CBT-i

provided asynchronous interaction with an insomnia specialist. Both groups had significant improvement in their ISI scores as well as in their sleep efficiency, latency, and quality. Patient satisfaction with treatment was similar in both groups.

Self-Directed Internet/App Cognitive Behavioral Therapy for Insomnia versus Placebo

A total of 303 adults were randomized to either I-CBT-i for 6 weeks with weekly modules or a Web-based placebo. Follow-up was maintained to 1 year. Individuals randomized to I-CBT-i had significant improvement in their ISI scores as well as sleep latency, which were maintained for a year after treatment.[27]

Meta-Analyses of Self-Directed Internet/App Cognitive Behavioral Therapy for Insomnia

A 2016 meta-analysis by Ye and colleagues[25] evaluated 15 randomized controlled studies comparing more than 1000 patients using I-CBT-i with 591 wait-list controls. Evaluation over 5 to 9 weeks found that I-CBT-i significantly decreased sleep-onset latency by 18.4 minutes, increased total sleep time by 22.3 minutes, increased sleep efficiency by 9.58%, and decreased the ISI by 5.88 points. A similar 2016 meta-analysis of 15 trials by Seyffert and colleagues[24] reached similar conclusions with the addition that Internet-delivered therapy performance was statistically no different from in-person therapy.

Tele-Cognitive Behavioral Therapy for Insomnia and Wearable Devices

As wearable devices such as smart watches and movement trackers become more commonplace, there is also significant potential to further track efficacy of and adherence to CBT-i. In 2017, Kang and colleagues[28] conducted a pilot study evaluating the efficacy of a wearable device in conjunction with use of a mobile application CBT-i program in 19 patients. Using the mobile app, patients in the study demonstrated improved sleep efficiency as measured both by sleep diaries and the wearable device, as well as improvement in ISI scores. No significant differences were noted between the individuals who did or not use the wearable devices.

Stepped-up Care Tele-Cognitive Behavioral Therapy for Insomnia

In light of the inherent advantages and disadvantages of the aforementioned approaches to tele-CBT-i, use of a "stepped care" framework in which patients begin with self-directed therapy and are "stepped-up" to fully directed therapy if nonresponsive, has been proposed to maximize efficacy and minimize costs.[29,30] Mohr and colleagues[30] examined this principle in a randomized noninferiority trial for depression by comparing Internet-based self-directed therapy stepped-up to telephone-administered fully directed therapy (tCBT) versus tCBT alone. Although the stepped-up model was more cost-effective and no less effective than tCBT, patient satisfaction was significantly lower in the stepped model. A recent study in young working adults in Japan comparted tailored I-BBT-i (performed by a computer algorithm) versus I-BBT-i, self-monitoring, and wait-list.[31] The tailored I-BBT-i was comparable with the I-BBT-i in reducing ISI scores, although the improvements in the tailored approaches were noted earlier. Drop-out rates were similar between the 2 groups. Of note, participants in this trial had mild insomnia, were young, and were employed. This population has been shown to do well with I CBT-i. Additional trials of "step-up" therapy targeting individuals with more severe insomnia and additional comorbidities are necessary.

Cognitive Behavioral Therapy for Insomnia and Pharmacologic Discontinuation

Although cognitive and behavioral-based therapies for insomnia are recommended as first-line therapy, there is a large segment of the population still using pharmacologic agents for the treatment of insomnia. Patients on pharmacologic therapy can take advantage of telehealth for insomnia to undergo CBT-i/BBT-i while at the same time titrating medications with the goal to discontinue pharmacotherapy. The current Big Bird trial is randomizing patients on benzodiazepines and z-drugs to either usual care or a blended model with access to a self-directed Internet module that provides education on their sleeping medication as well as cognitive behavioral techniques to assist the patient with deprescription.[32] A different and potential benefit of telemedicine, where CBT-i/BBT-i is not available, is the ability to assess efficacy, side effects, and appropriate use of pharmacologic therapy for insomnia. To date, not many studies are available in the field of insomnia pharmacotherapy discontinuation and use of telemedicine.

Telemedicine and Clinical Visit Telehealth-Insomnia: Pitfalls and Unanswered Questions

Despite a rapidly growing body of literature pointing to the importance and efficacy of I-CBT-i, the proliferation of unregulated applications leads to a number of limitations. Yu and colleagues[4] found that most currently available mobile applications for insomnia do not fully adhere to evidence-based CBT-i principles. Patients with severe insomnia tend to be underrepresented in these studies and thus efficacy in this important demographic may be underevaluated.[24] Many studies in the preceding meta-analyses also still incorporated regular face-to-face sessions, suggesting that self-directed therapy may best be a part of a blended or step care model. In a video-based self-directed study of 242 patients with breast cancer and insomnia, Savard and colleagues[33,34] found that although self-directed video-based treatment was effective, there was considerably more relapse insomnia in patients who did not receive individualized therapy. Leigh and colleagues[35] also raised additional concerns with regard to the regulation (or lack thereof) of I-CBT-i quality, efficacy, and protection of privacy. It is clear that more research is needed to better optimize and ensure quality delivery of self-directed CBT-i.

Although there has been a proliferation of data on the efficacy and utility of tele-CBT-I, many questions still need to be answered, among them are the following:

- What is the ideal level of therapist interaction for a specific patient to allow for optimal treatment results?
- What is the ideal modality for a specific patient to allow for optimal treatment results?
- Most studies predominantly include middle-aged, healthy, white women. What are the optimal treatment modalities for alternate patient populations, including those of different ethnicities and those with additional comorbidities?
- Can specialized programs be developed for individuals with varying levels of computer literacy?
- What unintended or adverse effects can occur with each modality outcomes?

CONCLUSION AND NEXT STEPS

There has been enormous progress in the evolution of tele-CBT-i with development of a variety of options from fully directed therapy with a provider to completely self-directed Internet or app-based CBT-i. Additional work is needed to personalize care based on patient characteristics, preference, and response to therapy.

DISCLOSURE

The authors have nothing to disclose.

REFERENCES

1. Dopheide JA. Insomnia overview: epidemiology, pathophysiology, diagnosis and monitoring, and nonpharmacologic therapy. Am J Manag Care 2020;26(4 Suppl):S76–84.
2. Singh J, Badr MS, Diebert W, et al. American Academy of Sleep Medicine (AASM) position paper for the use of telemedicine for the diagnosis and treatment of sleep disorders. J Clin Sleep Med 2015; 11(10):1187–98.
3. Sateia MJ, Buysse DJ, Krystal AD, et al. Clinical practice guideline for the pharmacologic treatment of chronic insomnia in adults: an American Academy of Sleep Medicine Clinical Practice Guideline. J Clin Sleep Med 2017;13(2):307–49.
4. Yu JS, Kuhn E, Miller KE, et al. Smartphone apps for insomnia: examining existing apps' usability and adherence to evidence-based principles for insomnia management. Transl Behav Med 2019; 9(1):110–9.
5. Qaseem A, Kansagara D, Forciea MA, et al. Management of chronic insomnia disorder in adults: a clinical practice guideline from the American College of Physicians. Ann Intern Med 2016;165(2): 125–33.
6. Management of insomnia disorder in adults: current state of the evidence | Effective Health Care Program. Available at: https://effectivehealthcare.ahrq. gov/products/insomnia/clinician. Accessed April 20, 2020.
7. Koffel E, Bramoweth AD, Ulmer CS. Increasing access to and utilization of cognitive behavioral therapy for insomnia (CBT-I): a narrative review. J Gen Intern Med 2018;33(6):955–62.
8. Ruskin PE, Silver-Aylaian M, Kling MA, et al. Treatment outcomes in depression: comparison of remote treatment through telepsychiatry to in-person treatment. Am J Psychiatry 2004;161(8):1471–6.
9. International Classification of Sleep Disorders. Third edition. Darien: American Academy of Sleep Medicine; 2014.
10. Mitchell MD, Gehrman P, Perlis M, et al. Comparative effectiveness of cognitive behavioral therapy for insomnia: a systematic review. BMC Fam Pract 2012;13:40.
11. (AASM) AAoSM. Brief behavioral treatment for insomnia. Available at: https://j2vjt3dnbra3 ps7ll1clb4q2-wpengine.netdna-ssl.com/wp-content/ uploads/2019/03/ProviderFS_BBTI_18.pdf. Accessed January 15, 2020.
12. Troxel WM, Germain A, Buysse DJ. Clinical management of insomnia with brief behavioral treatment (BBTI). Behav Sleep Med 2012;10(4):266–79.
13. Gunn HE, Tutek J, Buysse DJ. Brief behavioral treatment of insomnia. Sleep Med Clin 2019;14(2): 235–43.
14. Chakrabarti S. Usefulness of telepsychiatry: a critical evaluation of videoconferencing-based approaches. World J Psychiatry 2015;5(3): 286–304.
15. Hilty DM, Ferrer DC, Parish MB, et al. The effectiveness of telemental health: a 2013 review. Telemed J E Health 2013;19(6):444–54.
16. Shore JH, Yellowlees P, Caudill R, et al. Best practices in videoconferencing-based telemental health April 2018. Telemed J E Health 2018;24(11): 827–32.
17. Arnedt JT, Conroy D, Mooney A, et al. 0363 efficacy of cognitive behavioral therapy delivered via telemedicine vs. face-to-face: preliminary results from a randomized controlled non-inferiority trial. Sleep 2019;42:A148.
18. Gieselmann A, Pietrowsky R. The effects of brief chat-based and face-to-face psychotherapy for insomnia: a randomized waiting list controlled trial. Sleep Med 2019;61:63 72.
19. Blom K, Tarkian Tillgren H, Wiklund T, et al. Internet- vs. group-delivered cognitive behavior therapy for insomnia: a randomized controlled non-inferiority trial. Behav Res Ther 2015;70:47–55.
20. Gehrman P, Shah MT, Miles A, et al. Feasibility of group cognitive-behavioral treatment of insomnia delivered by clinical video telehealth. Telemed J E Health 2016;22(12):1041–6.
21. Dilgul M, McNamee P, Orfanos S, et al. Why do psychiatric patients attend or not attend treatment groups in the community: a qualitative study. PLoS One 2018;13(12):e0208448.
22. Holmqvist M, Vincent N, Walsh K. Web- vs. telehealth-based delivery of cognitive behavioral therapy for insomnia: a randomized controlled trial. Sleep Med 2014;15(2):187–95.
23. Strom L, Pettersson R, Andersson G. Internet-based treatment for insomnia: a controlled evaluation. J Consult Clin Psychol 2004;72(1):113–20.
24. Seyffert M, Lagisetty P, Landgraf J, et al. Internet-delivered cognitive behavioral therapy to treat insomnia: a systematic review and meta-analysis. PLoS One 2016;11(2):e0149139.
25. Ye YY, Chen NK, Chen J, et al. Internet-based cognitive-behavioural therapy for insomnia (ICBT-i): a meta-analysis of randomised controlled trials. BMJ Open 2016;6(11):e010707.
26. Zachariae R, Lyby MS, Ritterband LM, et al. Efficacy of internet-delivered cognitive-behavioral therapy for insomnia - a systematic review and meta-analysis of randomized controlled trials. Sleep Med Rev 2016; 30:1–10.
27. Ritterband LM, Thorndike FP, Ingersoll KS, et al. Effect of a web-based cognitive behavior therapy for insomnia intervention with 1-year follow-up: a randomized clinical trial. JAMA Psychiatry 2017;74(1): 68–75.

28. Kang SG, Kang JM, Cho SJ, et al. Cognitive behavioral therapy using a mobile application synchronizable with wearable devices for insomnia treatment: a pilot study. J Clin Sleep Med 2017; 13(4):633–40.

29. Espie CA. "Stepped care": a health technology solution for delivering cognitive behavioral therapy as a first line insomnia treatment. Sleep 2009;32(12): 1549–58.

30. Mohr DC, Lattie EG, Tomasino KN, et al. A randomized noninferiority trial evaluating remotely-delivered stepped care for depression using internet cognitive behavioral therapy (CBT) and telephone CBT. Behav Res Ther 2019;123:103485.

31. Okajima I, Akitomi J, Kajiyama I, et al. Effects of a tailored brief behavioral therapy application on insomnia severity and social disabilities among workers with insomnia in Japan: a randomized clinical trial. JAMA Netw Open 2020;3(4):e202775.

32. Coteur K, Van Nuland M, Vanmeerbeek M, et al. Effectiveness of a blended care programme for the discontinuation of benzodiazepine use for sleeping problems in primary care: study protocol of a cluster randomised trial, the Big Bird trial. BMJ Open 2020; 10(2):e033688.

33. Savard J, Ivers H, Savard MH, et al. Is a video-based cognitive behavioral therapy for insomnia as efficacious as a professionally administered treatment in breast cancer? Results of a randomized controlled trial. Sleep 2014;37(8):1305–14.

34. Savard J, Ivers H, Savard MH, et al. Long-term effects of two formats of cognitive behavioral therapy for insomnia comorbid with breast cancer. Sleep 2016;39(4):813–23.

35. Leigh S, Ouyang J, Mimnagh C. Effective? Engaging? Secure? Applying the ORCHA-24 framework to evaluate apps for chronic insomnia disorder. Evid Based Ment Health 2017;20(4):e20.

Current and Future Roles of Consumer Sleep Technologies in Sleep Medicine

Cathy Goldstein, MD, MS

KEYWORDS

• Consumer sleep technology • Actigraphy • Remote patient monitoring

KEY POINTS

- Consumer sleep technologies are products marketed directly to consumers for the purpose of tracking sleep and can be coarsely grouped into wearables, nearables, and stand-alone mobile apps.
- Consumer sleep technology is the system of sensors within the device and the associated mobile application and cloud-based platform for data management and visualization.
- These technologies include sensors that measure motion, heart rate, oximetry, respiration, temperature, neuronal activity, and other parameters to differentiate sleep from wake, determine sleep stages, and identify other relevant sleep metrics.
- Some consumer sleep technologies provide feedback to the user through mobile application delivered behavioral recommendations or acoustic or physical intervention.
- Clinical adoption of consumer sleep technologies is limited by lack of validation studies in the peer-reviewed literature and absent clearance by the US Food and Drug Administration.

INTRODUCTION

The world market for wearable devices is expected to exceed $60 billion by 2025 and the health care industry is forecasted as the greatest end-user of wearable mobile technologies.[1] Approximately one-third of the US population reports regularly tracking their sleep with use of smartphones or other digital technologies[2] and, not surprisingly, sleep medicine providers have witnessed the permeation of consumer products into everyday clinical practice.

Our field is well-positioned to benefit from products marketed directly to patients and used in the home owing to the following paradox present in sleep medicine. Sleep disorders are chronic, and symptoms typically result from persistent, daily exposure to disturbances in sleep quality and/or duration. However, the cornerstone for diagnostic testing and gold-standard for sleep measurement is the polysomnogram (PSG) which, owing to the requirement of a sleep laboratory, technicians, and monitoring of multiple physiologic parameters, is typically restricted to the assessment of sleep over 1 or 2 nights.[3]

Objective, longitudinal sleep measurement in the clinical setting is currently available through the use of US Food and Drug Administration (FDA) cleared actigraphy, which uses wrist-worn accelerometry devices that measure movement to estimate sleep. Actigraphy is well-accepted by the medical and research communities, given the large body of peer-reviewed evidence has assessed sleep estimation accuracy against PSG[4–6]; however, significant inadequacies limit usefulness, such as expense, the requirement of a trained member of the sleep team to set up the device and recover the data, and lack of easy integration between actigraphy software and the

University of Michigan Sleep Disorders Center, 1500 East Medical Center Drive, Med Inn C728, Ann Arbor, MI 48109, USA
E-mail address: cathygo@med.umich.edu

Sleep Med Clin 15 (2020) 391–408
https://doi.org/10.1016/j.jsmc.2020.05.001
1556-407X/20/© 2020 Elsevier Inc. All rights reserved.

electronic medical record or other digital health data sources. Additionally, reimbursement for recording and interpretation is unlikely despite a Current Procedural Technology code. Therefore, historically, despite the relevance for the accurate diagnosis and efficient management of sleep disorders,[7,8] longitudinal, objective monitoring of sleep duration, quantity, and timing has not been routinely incorporated into clinical practice. Consequently, sleep providers frequently rely on self-report sleep measures, which are often inaccurate or incomplete.[9]

Consumer sleep technologies (CSTs) have presented a tempting solution to the problem of ambulatory sleep tracking given ease of use, widespread availability, low cost, and opportunity for integration with other health technology products; however, minimal validation and lack of transparency in regard to acquisition and analysis of data has previously tempered the enthusiasm for their use in medicine. However, this paradigm is beginning to shift as initial studies demonstrate the potential clinical usefulness of commercially available products in other specialties.[10]

The unprecedented speed of technological advance is expected to rapidly expand the number of consumer-marketed products that analyze, store, and distill vast amounts of health-related data. Because sleep health is marked by the convergence of behavior and biology, our field stands to greatly benefit from such tools that lie on the interface of clinical and consumer technology. The data transmission capabilities of CSTs and widespread ownership by patients are particularly well-suited to incorporation in a telemedicine workflow because data can be collected and viewed independent of an in-person exchange. The sleep data derived from appropriately vetted CSTs could provide valuable adjunct information about sleep patterns and characteristics of the home sleep environment for both synchronous and asynchronous virtual health.

This article describes the landscape of CSTs, but is not a comprehensive review of specific devices (examples can be found in **Tables 1** and **2**). Instead, mechanisms that underlie the acquisition and analysis of the data derived from different classes of products, framework of the validation process to assess accuracy, potential use cases, and future applications are discussed.

CONSUMER SLEEP TECHNOLOGIES: THE BASICS

CSTs are coarsely grouped into 3 categories: wearables, nearables, and mobile applications (apps) that function without a separate associated device.

Both wearables and nearables are associated with companion mobile apps and cloud-based platforms for data analysis, management, and viewing. CST will be used to reference the sleep estimation system (sensors plus data management methods) as a whole. Examples of various CSTs can be found in **Tables 1** and **2**.

Wearable Sensors

Wrist-worn (and ring) consumer sleep technologies
The large-scale adoption of sleep tracking technologies directly to consumers is owed to wrist-worn CSTs and such devices continue to dominate the CST marketplace. Initially, wrist-worn CSTs recorded only movement; however, current generation devices are multisensory, and typically record motion and heart rate; sometimes temperature and skin conductance; and more recently, oxygen saturation.[11]

The motion data acquired by wrist-worn CST are obtained via an accelerometer, which uses a piezoelectric sensor that produces a voltage signal in response to movement.[12] Such sensors are now miniaturized by microelectromechanical system technology and rapid advances in accelerometer development have allowed for increased memory and battery capacity, wide acceleration range, and low cost.[13] Acceleration is typically recorded in 3 axes (triaxial) and expressed in units of g ($1g = 9.8$ m/s^2), but then further processed into count data.[12]

Pulse rate is determined at the dorsal aspect of the wrist through photoplethysmography (PPG), an optical technique that quantifies blood volume changes, which has been validated to accurately measure heart rate in multiple contexts.[14,15] PPG data are also used as surrogates for other values typically derived from electrocardiogram (such as heart rate variability).[14,15] Of note, the usefulness of consumer-available PPG measured at the dorsum of the wrist is underscored by FDA clearance of a mobile app that analyzes PPG signal acquired by the Apple Watch for over-the-counter use to evaluate for irregular heart rhythms.[16] In some CSTs, algorithms are applied to PPG heart rate to indirectly estimate respiratory rate based on the known relationship between heart rate and respiration.[17]

PPG is also a well-accepted method to measure blood oxygen saturation and in the clinical context is typically positioned on the fingertip.[18] Recently, this feature has been activated in certain wrist-worn CSTs such that blood oxygen saturations can be extracted from the PPG sensor at the dorsum of the wrist.[19]

Table 1
Examples of wearable CST

Manufacturer	Model	Motion/ Activity	HR	POx	TEMP	EEG	Other Features
Wrist-worn CST							
Withings	Steel HR	✓	✓				
	Move	✓					
	Move ECG	✓	✓				ECG; Afib detection
	Pulse HR	✓	✓				
Garmin[a]	MARQ Adventurer	✓	✓	✓	✓		
	Tactix delta	✓	✓	✓	✓		
	Fenix 6	✓	✓	✓	✓		
	Fenix 5x	✓	✓	✓	✓		
	D2 Delta PX	✓	✓	✓	✓		
	Vivosmart 4	✓	✓	✓			
	Venu	✓	✓	✓	✓		
	First Avenger	✓	✓	✓	✓		
FitBit	Versa 2	✓	✓				
	Versa Lite	✓	✓				
	Ionic	✓	✓				
	Charge 4	✓	✓				
	Inspire	✓					
	Inspire HR	✓	✓				
	Charge 3	✓	✓				
	Ace 2	✓					
Whoop	Whoop Strap 3.0	✓	✓		✓		
Philips	Philips Health Watch	✓	✓				
EverSleep	EverSleep	✓	✓	✓			POx worn on finger
Polar	A370	✓	✓				
	M430	✓	✓				
Misfit	Vapor	✓	✓				
	Command	✓					
	Path	✓					
Biostrap	Biostrap	✓	✓	✓			Add on chest, armband and leg strap; leg movement monitoring
Lookee Tech	Lookee Wrist sleep monitor	✓	✓	✓			POx within ring
Ring CST							
Oura	Oura ring	✓	✓		✓		
Thim	Thim ring	✓					Vibratory stimuli for intensive sleep retraining
Lookee Tech	Lookee Ring Pro	✓	✓	✓			Vibration alert for low oxygen
Headband CST							
Dreem	Dreem2	✓	✓	✓		✓	Slow wave promotion

(continued on next page)

Table 1
(continued)

Manufacturer	Model	Motion/ Activity	HR	POx	TEMP	EEG	Other Features
Muse	Muse S	✓	✓	✓		✓	Guided meditation with biofeedback
Philips	SmartSleep Deep Sleep					✓	Slow wave promotion
Eye mask CST							
Dreamlight	Dreamlight Pro	✓	✓				Genetic testing; light guided breathing; surround sound
Neuroon	Neuroon	✓	✓	✓	✓	✓	+EOG, biofeedback for meditation
Other CST							
Kokoon	KoKoon	✓				✓	Headphones, relaxation techniques and music
Beddr	Beddr sleep Tuner	✓	✓	✓			Forehead sensor

Parameters measured acquired from those listed on manufacturer web sites; other metrics may be available.

Abbreviations: Afib, atrial fibrillation; ECG, electrocardiogram; EEG, electroencephalogram; EOG, electrooculogram; HR, heart rate; POx, pulse oximetry; TEMP, temperature.

[a] Advanced sleep monitoring is available on 33 models; only a sample listed here.

Ring CSTs comprise a much smaller portion of the wearable CST market compared with wrist-worn devices. Like wrist-worn devices, ring CSTs use accelerometry to measure movement and PPG to measure pulse and derived values. One of the few ring devices available also measures temperature[20] and others are novel given the ability to provide a vibratory stimulus for the purpose of intensive sleep retraining for insomnia[21] or as an alert to low oxygen levels and apneas (see **Table 1**).

The incorporation of accelerometer and PPG sensors into wrist-worn and ring CSTs permit 24-hour use. However, some emerging CSTs focus on PPG and accelerometer data collection primarily during the nocturnal sleep period and, therefore, can leverage other physical locations for sensor placement such as the forehead, wrist and finger combined, or over the eyes (see **Table 1**).

For a comprehensive review of accelerometer and PPG sensors as well as other sensors incorporated into wearable CST; such as those that monitor temperature, skin conductance, respiration, and light, see de Zambotti and colleagues.[11]

Dry electroencephalogram headbands

The explosion of wearable wrist-worn CSTs and concept of the "quantified self" in general was actually heralded by the 2009 introduction of a dry electroencephalogram (EEG) headband that estimated sleep and timed an alarm to promote wake up out of lighter sleep stages. However, the company was defunct by 2013; unfortunately, after multiple validation studies of the device's performance were conducted and published.[22] Dry EEG headbands do not require adhesive to affix EEG sensors and, therefore, allow EEG recording to take place at home. Dry EEG headbands have reemerged in the CST marketplace and the current iterations often include closed-loop systems, for example, the identification of slow waves and augmentation by acoustic stimuli.[23] A newer technology combines EEG with electrooculogram, PPG, and accelerometer sensors within an eye mask (see **Table 1**), although peer-reviewed data have yet to describe whether such an approach results in more accurate performance.

Table 2
Examples of nearable CST

| Manufacturer | Model | Measures | | Other Features |
		User	Sleep Environment	
Noncontact bedside nearable				
ResMed and SleepScore labs	S+/SleepScoreMax	Sleep stages	Ambient light, noise, and temperature	
Under-the-mattress nearables				
Apple	Beddit	Sleep, heart rate, breathing, snoring	Ambient temperature, humidity	
Withings	Sleep Sensing & Home Automation Pad	Sleep stages, heart rate, snoring, 'breathing disturbances'		Integrates with smart home devices
Sleep Number	Sleep Number Bed with Sleep IQ	Restful and restless sleep, heart rate, respiratory rate		Within mattress; warms feet to help induce sleep
EmFit	EmFit QS	Sleep stages, heart rate, respiratory rate, movement		Focus on HRV for recovery
Other nearables				
Somnox	Sleep robot	Breathing		Item held during sleep that monitors and synchronizes breathing

Parameters measured acquired from those listed on manufacturer web sites; other metrics may be available.
Abbreviation: HRV, heart rate variability.

Nearable Sensors

Bedside

Noncontact bedside radiofrequency biomotion sensors (see **Table 2**) are desirable to consumers interested in tracking their sleep without wearing any additional devices.[24–26] Noncontact bedside radiofrequency biomotion sensors are placed at the bedside and measure movement with ultralow power radiofrequency waves and use the premise that during sleep, most detected movement should be related to respiratory effort.[25]

Under the mattress

Under-the-mattress CSTs are based on the static charge-sensitive bed, which was developed approximately 40 years ago and measures ballistocardiography (the visual representation of body movement owing to cardiac expulsion of blood

into the arteries) and respiratory and body motion.[27] The static charge-sensitive bed uses metal plates placed under a mattress.[27] Movement from the individual in the bed creates a charge and the potential difference between the 2 plates is analyzed to determine cardiac and respiratory measures.[27] Additionally, modeling of these data predicts sleep stages, and in the initial description in the 1981 *American Journal of Physiology*, the static charge-sensitive bed was offered as a potential future alternative to "very expensive and troublesome" sleep studies.[27] The more modern iterations of under-the-mattress CSTs (see **Table 2**) use a thin flexible force sensor to measure ballistocardiography and derived sleep measures, and one device also monitors temperature and humidity.[28]

Mobile Applications

A vast number of standalone mobile apps are available that claim to track sleep or respiration during sleep, and even provide coaching or intervention.[29,30] Data acquisition is often through sensors native to the smartphone that the app is downloaded on (eg, sleep tracking with the embedded accelerometer or snore assessment via the microphone). However, some apps acquire data through direct input by the user, or indirectly with analysis of smart phone use.[29–31] The rapid turnover of such sleep targeted apps precludes a comprehensive review here, although apps with the purpose of sleep tracking, alarms, obstructive sleep apnea diagnosis/treatment, and interventions targeted at insomnia have been described and, overall, are well-accepted by consumers.[29,30]

Although the ability of standalone mobile apps to accurately estimate sleep and respiratory parameters remains unclear, behavioral interventions delivered by apps have demonstrated usefulness in the management of various sleep disorders. Patient facing mobile apps allow for digital cognitive behavioral therapy for insomnia (see Caleb Hsieh and colleagues' article, "Telemedicine and the Management of Insomnia," in this issue) obstructive sleep apnea self-management (see Sharon Schutte-Rodin's article, "Telehealth, Telemedicine, and Obstructive Sleep Apnea," in this issue), and sleep extension.[32]

Data Processing and Management

The data acquired by sensors housed in wearable and nearable devices and smartphones are sent to a device specific app and often channeled to a cloud-based server. Algorithms are applied to these data to distinguish sleep from wake and often designate sleep stages (**Fig. 1**).

The algorithms in the sleep scoring software packages associated with traditional, clinical-grade actigraphy are typically based on weighted sums applied to activity count data.[33–35] However, the sleep estimation algorithms used by CSTs are

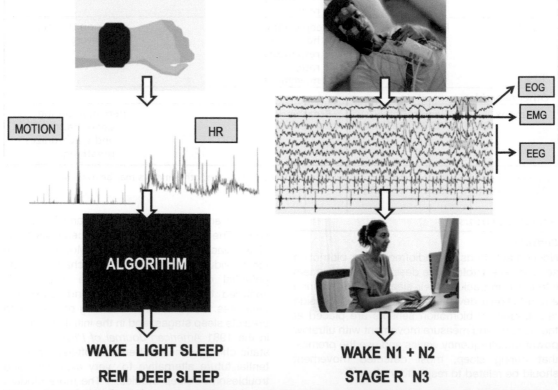

Fig. 1. CST and PSG, from data acquisition to sleep metrics. CSTs and PSGs measure different physiologic processes, which are analyzed in different ways to predict sleep stages using different terminologies. For example, a wrist-worn CST might record motion and heart rate (HR) data from triaxial accelerometer and PPG sensors and then "black box" algorithms are applied to these data to differentiate wake from sleep and estimate light, deep, and REM sleep for the user. For the purposes of sleep staging, PSG records electrooculogram (EOG), electromyogram (EMG), and electroencephalogram (EEG), and these signals are analyzed by a registered polysomnographic technologist and labeled as wake, N1, N2, N3, and stage R sleep. N1, NREM 1; N2, NREM 2; N3, NREM 3; R, REM.

considered 'black box' because they are not typically disclosed by manufacturers and use unknown features derived from motion, heart rate, and other physiologic data points. Few peer-reviewed publications have applied researcher-developed algorithms to signal acquired with off-the-shelf CSTs and compared their performance with PSG.[36–39] Such methodology offers a more scientifically rigorous, transparent approach, particularly if the code for such analysis methods is disclosed.[39] The use of heart rate variability (from PPG) as a feature in sleep-staging algorithms seems to be a powerful feature in the analysis of data from CST sensors.[37,40] As the body of literature regarding modeling signal from CST sensors grows, other physiologic features and mathematically derived parameters such as circadian estimates[39] and

models of the sleep homeostat may continue to improve sleep staging performance.

A nuanced but highly relevant component of the transformation of raw data acquired from CST sensors to summary sleep metrics is the designation of the time in bed window.[41] Sleep estimation algorithms are not applied continuously to 24-hour data and, therefore, accurate differentiation of sleep and wake hinges on the correct window to deploy such classifiers (**Fig. 2**). Previously, older iterations of CST required users to actively designate the window within which sleep was attempted, but to make sleep tracking completely passive; the time in bed window is now automatically designated (with unclear accuracy).

After analysis, summary sleep data are displayed to the individual via the app user interface and various, manufacturer specific terminology

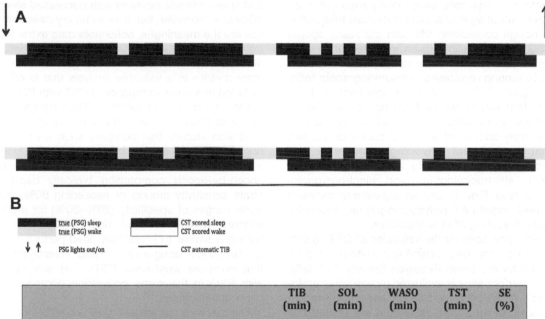

	TIB (min)	SOL (min)	WASO (min)	TST (min)	SE (%)
PSG sleep measures (ground truth)	480	20	160	300	62.5%
A- CST sleep measures, manual TIB (synchronized with PSG lights on/off)	480	10	60	410	85.4%
B-CST sleep measures, automated/passive TIB (unverified CST algorithm)	370	0	50	320	86.4%

Fig. 2. Impact of manual versus automated TIB on CST summary sleep metrics given epoch-by-epoch sensitivity of 97% and specificity of 33%. A theoretic validation study that compares a CST with PSG records 480 minutes time in bed, and PSG (ground truth) sleep duration of 300 minutes and wakefulness of 180 minutes. Epoch-by-epoch comparison reveals that the CST designates 290 minutes of true sleep correctly (sensitivity of 97%) and 60 minutes of true wake correctly (specificity of 33%), but misclassifies 120 minutes of wake as sleep and 10 minutes of sleep as wakefulness. Summary sleep metrics quantified by the CST on the same night differ based on how TIB is defined (set manually by synchronizing the CST TIB with PSG lights on/lights off [A] vs use of the CST automated TIB algorithm [B], which is how the CST would be used in real life). TIB, time in bed; SOL, sleep onset latency; WASO, wake after sleep onset; TST, total sleep time; SE, sleep efficiency.

(with and without corresponding established clinical equivalents) are used to describe sleep parameters. Although the precise measures reported vary between manufacturer platforms, the following are often quantified: bedtime, wake-up time, total sleep time (TST), wake time, light sleep, deep sleep, and REM sleep. Sleep quality may be indicated by terms such as "restless sleep" and "sleep disturbances." Of note, CST specifically geared toward athletes or other industries may have web-based platforms that present the data in aggregate form to a trainer or other staff member responsible for determining fitness for duty.

VALIDATION
Sleep Scoring

For a CST to be considered an acceptable method to estimate sleep, comparison of algorithm output against scored PSG must take place. Although considered the gold standard, scored PSG is not infallible given imperfect inter-rater reliability, with overall percent agreement around 80% among registered polysomnographic technologists.[42,43] Therefore, the appraisal of statistics that reflect the performance of automated estimation of sleep from a CST compared with manually scored PSG should take into account that (1) different physiologic properties are recorded (eg, heart rate and motion data vs EEG, electrooculogram, and electromyogram data) (see **Fig. 1**) and (2) agreement between expert registered polysomnographic technologists in scoring PSG is imperfect.

Best practices for the validation of CST against PSG are described in detail in a white paper published by the Sleep Research Society .[44] Briefly, CST performance is evaluated by validation protocols where PSG is recorded in individuals simultaneously using a CST. PSG data are scored and time synchronized with the CST output such that the same 30-second time intervals (epochs) can be compared (**Fig. 3**), although measures to reconcile data of different time scales (eg, 1-minute CST output) have been described.[45] From this epoch-by-epoch analysis, sensitivity, specificity, and accuracy can be reported.

Sensitivity refers to the fraction of PSG sleep epochs designated correctly as sleep by the CST and specificity refers to the fraction of PSG wake epochs designated correctly as wake by the CST (see **Fig. 3**). Owing to reliance, at least in part, of CSTs on movement to distinguish sleep from wake, specificity is often much lower than sensitivity given nonmoving wakefulness is frequently misclassified as sleep. Therefore, CSTs typically overestimate TST and underestimate wakefulness in comparison with PSG,[44,45] although this is not always the case.[20,46–48]

Accuracy refers to the fraction of scored PSG epochs correctly designated by the CST and may be misleading in healthy individuals given most of the overnight period is spent asleep; therefore, even if a CST algorithm arbitrarily scores every single 30-second epoch as sleep, if sleep efficiency is high, accuracy will also be deceptively high. Similarly, summary sleep metrics over the course of the night, such as TST and wake after sleep onset, compared between a CST and PSG should not be used as a sole measure of performance, because these measures may be statistically similar in individuals with high sleep efficiency but discrepant in individuals with poor quality sleep. Therefore, the amount of sleep misclassified by a CST of a given reported sensitivity and specificity will increase with decreased sleep efficiency. However, because summary sleep metrics are the meaningful, actionable data extracted from CSTs, the use of a Bland-Altman plot to visualize discrepancies and direction of bias of summary metrics is a valuable analysis that is often included in studies comparing a CST with PSG.

The performance of specific CSTs is beyond the scope of this article. A comprehensive review of validation studies that compare wrist-worn (and ring) CST to PSG are can be found in de Zambotti and colleagues.[45] Validation studies that use epoch-by-epoch comparison typically demonstrate sensitivity around or exceeding 90%, but wider ranges of specificity (20%–80%) for multisensory wrist-worn (and ring) CST.[44,45] This finding is similar to historically cited performance for traditional actigraphy,[4–6] and investigations that compare wrist-worn CSTs and actigraphy with PSG in the same population demonstrate minimal differences.[44]

The currently marketed dry EEG headbands do not have sleep–wake performance reported in the peer-reviewed literature; however, validation studies that used a previously available dry EEG headband device reported sensitivity of 97.6% and specificity of 56.1%[49] and overall agreement around 90%.[50]

An under-the-mattress CST, although based on the verified principle of ballistocardiography, significantly underestimated wake after sleep onset and overestimated TST.[28] In contrast, an FDA-cleared under-the-mattress sensor detected sleep with a sensitivity and specificity of 92.5% and 80.4%, respectively.[51]

The few validation studies of noncontact bedside nearable devices also demonstrated a bias toward overestimating TST in both healthy

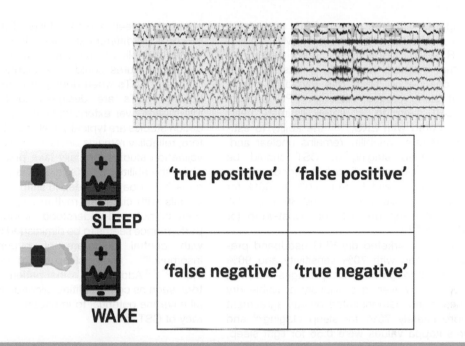

Fig. 3. Epoch-by-epoch comparison between CST and PSG. Performance metrics of CST during an epoch-by-epoch comparison with PSG can be conceptualized with use of a traditional 4 × 4 table. Typically, such tables are used to compare the disease prediction capability of a new test to gold standard in a population with and without disease who undergo testing with both modalities. In the case of CSTs, the new test is the CST and the gold standard is PSG scored by a registered polysomnographic technologist. However, the population is not individuals, but time-synchronized epochs during recording of both CST and PSG, and the condition of interest is the sleep state (positive) versus wake state (negative). Therefore, the sensitivity of a CST is the fraction of PSG sleep epochs (true positive + false negative) that were correctly designated as sleep by the CST (true positive). Specificity is the fraction of PSG wake epochs (true negative + false positive) that were correctly designated as wake by the CST (true negative).

subjects[24,26] and those with sleep-disordered breathing.[25] When epoch-by-epoch comparisons were performed with use of noncontact bedside nearable devices, sensitivity was cited at 87% to 88%, whereas specificity ranged more widely at 50% to 73%, although different devices, software versions, and patient populations preclude direct comparison.[24,25]

The capacity of standalone mobile apps to differentiate sleep from wake is highly variable; one investigation demonstrated similar performance to traditional actigraphy in healthy individuals (sensitivity nearing 90% and specificity around 50%),[52] whereas others demonstrated marked misclassification of nonmoving wakefulness as sleep with significant overestimation of TST[46] or completely absent correlation in app-derived sleep metrics with PSG.[53] To isolate

sensor fidelity from algorithm performance, investigators applied a well-validated model used to estimate sleep from wrist actigraphy to accelerometry data from a smartphone.[36] Participants in the study simultaneously wore actigraphs, so that the output of the same algorithms applied to different sources of motion data could be compared on the same night. Satisfactory agreement was noted for TST, wake after sleep onset, and sleep efficiency, but not for sleep onset latency.[36] Therefore, with access to raw motion data from smartphones, well-validated algorithms traditionally applied to actigraphy have the potential to provide reasonable sleep estimates.

Sleep staging

In addition to sleep–wake differentiation, CSTs often classify sleep as light, deep, and REM, which is compared with the scored PSG equivalents NREM1 + NREM2 (N1 + N2), NREM3 (N3),and stage R sleep, respectively. Sleep staging by CSTs that measure heart rate is based on the known changes in heart rate variability during different sleep stages. Although PPG sensors within CST seem to accurately estimate heart rate compared with EKG,[54,55] the ability to estimate heart rate variability remains unclear and, therefore, sleep staging by CST should be approached cautiously. Epoch-by-epoch agreement has ranged widely, from 60% to 80% for N1+N2, 40% to 70% for N3, and 30% to 70% for stage R sleep derived from wrist-worn (or ring) CST.[20,56–58]

A currently marketed dry EEG headband predicted N3 sleep with 70% sensitivity and 90% specificity; although other sleep stages were not reported.[23] However, a previously available dry EEG headband demonstrated overall agreement of approximately 75% for sleep staging[50] and Cohen's kappa values were 0.56 for light sleep, 0.70 for deep sleep, and 0.67 for REM sleep in a different investigation of the same device.[49]

The peer-reviewed literature contains few studies that compare the sleep staging capability of nearable CSTs with PSG. A noncontact bedside nearable demonstrated 60%, 65% to 68%, 52% to 61%, and 62% agreement with PSG epochs staged as N1, N2, N3, and stage R sleep,[24] whereas an under-the-bed sensor demonstrated poor agreement with PSG staged sleep (Cohen's kappa = 0.1).[28] Standalone mobile apps have demonstrated minimal correlation between app quantified sleep stages and PSG.[30]

CST also frequently report sleep scores or other numerical metrics without disclosure of the definition or components that the values are calculated from and therefore, relevance or validity remains unclear.

The quality of the sensors and algorithms used by a manufacturer are the primary contributors to in-laboratory performance of CSTs compared with PSG; however, additional factors interfere with generalization of cited CST performance in the laboratory to the ambulatory setting. By design, validation protocols artificially set the window for time in bed in which CST and PSG sleep scoring is compared (see **Fig. 2**). Therefore, the performance cited for a CST may not translate to real-life use of the device, where sleep tracking is typically passive without user input, and deployment of sleep scoring algorithms depends on the automatic detection of the time in bed window (see **Fig. 2**). As such, the accuracy of reported sleep metrics is contingent on both the correct identification of when the patient is in bed

attempting sleep and the ability of the algorithm to correctly differentiate sleep from wake.[41] To further complicate matters, device position and technical failures could also change the performance of CSTs when deployed in real life. Additionally, CSTs are designed to collect sleep information over extensive time periods, but validation studies are typically limited to 1 night; therefore, reliability remains unclear. Similarly, because validation studies typically take place during the night, the ability of CSTs to estimate sleep during naps[58,59] or daytime sleep in shift workers or individuals with circadian rhythm sleep–wake disorders is not well-understood. Importantly, CST performance seems to be diminished in individuals with central disorders of hypersomnia,[57,58] insomnia,[60] and sleep-disordered breathing.[46,61–63] Additionally, other patient-specific factors, such as comorbidities, alcohol use, and age, all have the potential to impact the real-life accuracy of CST.[44]

RESPIRATORY PARAMETERS

Wrist-worn CST have recently opened up the capability to measure and report oximetry values; however, accuracy remains unknown. Oximetry values from a wrist-worn FDA cleared device have been validated[64]; whether this can extend to PPG housed in CSTs is unclear, however.

Wearable CST that use PPG can also report the respiratory rate if appropriate algorithms are applied to HR data; however, accuracy is not well-defined. Recently, a bias of 1.8% and precision error of 6.7% were found when respiratory rate estimates from a wrist-worn CST marketed to athletes was compared with the respiratory rate from respiratory inductance plethysmography during PSG.[65]

The capacity of wearable CST to measure oximetry and heart rate–derived respiratory metrics suggest that these devices might soon report apnea–hypopnea indices, but validation studies are not currently available. However, the capability of nearable CST to estimate the apnea–hypopnea index (AHI) is better defined. Using an AHI threshold of 15 per hour, under-the-mattress CSTs were able to identify obstructive sleep apnea with sensitivities ranging from 72% to 89% and specificities ranging from 70% to 91%.[66–68] Using the same AHI threshold, a noncontact bedside nearable appropriately classified obstructive sleep apnea with a sensitivity of 90% and a specificity of 92%.[69]

Many mobile apps claim to detect snoring through the smartphone microphone, although accuracy has varied widely.[30] Other apps have aimed to identify patients with obstructive sleep apnea. With the use of an AHI cutoff of 15 events per hour, 1 mobile app demonstrated a sensitivity of 70% and a specificity 94% in detecting obstructive sleep apnea compared with PSG, and another device had an accuracy of 92% compared with home testing.[70,71]

REGULATION AND GUIDELINES

The devices discussed here fall under the designation of "wellness" products and do not have FDA clearance; therefore, the American Academy of Sleep Medicine has recommended against the use of CSTs for the diagnosis or treatment of sleep disorders.[72] However, the distinction between diagnostic tools and wellness products may become increasingly more difficult, particularly now that many wrist-worn CSTs offer oximetry readings.

In response to the new regulatory challenges posed by rapidly evolving health technologies, the FDA set forth a Digital Health Innovation Action Plan that included a Software Pre-certification (Pre-cert) Pilot Program to regulate software as a medical device (SaMD). The FDA defines SaMD as "software intended to be used for one or more medical purposes that perform these purposes without being part of a hardware medical device."[73]

In addition to use with traditional medical platforms (eg, a software program that augments a radiologist's interpretation), SaMD can run on commercial off-the-shelf platforms.[73] Therefore, if a CST manufacturer pursued FDA clearance, the SaMD Pre-cert program would provide the pipeline for approval. The SaMD Pre-cert Program plans to provide a precertified designation to manufacturers of software and digital health technologies that demonstrate a culture of quality and organizational excellence.[73] Precertified manufacturers will be permitted to release SaMD into the market in an expedited manner after a streamlined review.[73] Continued monitoring will determine the real-word safety, effectiveness, and performance of the approved SaMD.[73] The 9 companies selected for the SaMD Pre-cert Pilot Program include developers of CST (eg, FitBit)[73] and, therefore, this program has future implications for the integration of CSTs into the practice of sleep medicine.

USE CASES
Actigraphy as a Precedent

The most immediate potential integration of appropriately verified CSTs into clinical sleep medicine is for the longitudinal sleep estimates historically attained with actigraphy. The International Classification of Sleep Disorders, 3rd edition, recommends actigraphy as part of the diagnostic evaluation in several disorders.[7] For suspected central disorders of hypersomnolence, use of actigraphy is recommended for at least 1 week to ensure adequate sleep duration before in-laboratory assessment with PSG and multiple sleep latency testing, document 24-hour sleep duration of longer than 660 minutes in certain cases of idiopathic hypersomnia, and identify chronic, recurrent sleep restriction in insufficient sleep syndrome.[7] Sleep estimation with actigraphy is also recommended to evaluate sleep–wake timing in circadian rhythm sleep–wake disorders; for at least 7 days in suspected delayed sleep–wake phase disorder, advanced sleep–wake phase disorder, irregular sleep–wake rhythm disorder, and shift work disorder, and for at least 14 days to visualize the nonentrained rest–activity pattern of non–24-hour sleep–wake rhythm disorder.[7]

After systematic review of the available peer-reviewed literature, a task force of the American Academy of Sleep Medicine confirmed the aforementioned rationale for use of actigraphy before PSG and multiple sleep latency testing, and in the evaluation suspected insufficient sleep syndrome and circadian rhythm sleep–wake disorder. Additionally, the task force identified the ability of actigraphy to estimate sleep parameters in insomnia and approximate sleep duration during home sleep apnea testing as part of an integrated device.[8] Sleep parameters obtained through actigraphy also reflected treatment response in insomnia, circadian rhythm sleep–wake disorder, and insufficient sleep syndrome.

The task force's recommendations were predicated on work that demonstrated that, for certain sleep parameters, actigraphy provides objective data that is often unique from patient-reported sleep logs. Therefore, a CST with accuracy that matches or exceeds a set benchmark considered acceptable for clinical use would have a variety of already identified applications.

New Applications

Although the most obvious role of CSTs in clinical sleep medicine would be to replace traditional clinical-grade actigraphy, CSTs have unique attributes such as widespread acceptance by patients, lower cost, ownership by the patient not the health system, long-term and continuous patterns of use, the ability to recharge easily, wireless and near real-time data transmission, and the capacity to integrate with other apps and health technologies. Such characteristics confer possibilities that transcend the use cases noted for actigraphy. Additionally, nearables, which do not have a clinical equivalent already in use, could add novel, valuable data to the clinical sleep evaluation, such as information about the home sleep environment (lighting, ambient temperature, air quality, and sound) and improve adherence to sleep tracking and subsequent interventions given truly passive use.

Data-driven circadian rhythm prediction

Whereas actigraphy is typically used to identify sleep and wake periods in suspected circadian rhythm sleep–wake disorder such that the abnormal pattern of sleep-wake timing can be visualized, mathematical modeling of 24-hour motion signal for days to weeks can quantify circadian properties of the rest–activity rhythm. Traditionally, cosinor analysis has been applied to actigraphy to estimate acrophase, mesor, period, and amplitude of the rest–activity rhythm; however, this analysis is poorly suited to patterns that change over time and a growing field of research that uses nonparametric, data-driven methods is likely to reveal more accurate techniques to capture circadian rhythmicity.[74,75] However, these techniques have not yet been incorporated into clinical use. When appropriately vetted, such models may be well-suited for an analysis of CST data to estimate circadian phase.

Off-positive airway pressure sleep time

Continuous positive airway pressure (CPAP) is the first line of therapy for obstructive sleep apnea, the most common disorder treated in sleep medicine. CPAP machines collect data regarding use, mask fit, and respiratory parameters determined from airflow assessment within the device. Such data have been integrated into the sleep medicine clinic encounter to augment the management of patients with obstructive sleep apnea.

Treatment of obstructive sleep apnea with CPAP is expected to resolve symptoms attributable to sleep-disordered breathing like sleep disruption and excessive daytime sleepiness. Additionally, because obstructive sleep apnea increases cardiovascular risk, treatment with CPAP is hypothesized to mitigate this risk, although randomized controlled trials have returned negative findings regarding benefit.[76,77] One obvious contribution to null findings is decreased patient adherence to CPAP, which is easily tracked with CPAP-generated use data. However, Thomas and Bianchi[78] proposed that the effectiveness of CPAP should be considered not only in absolute

hours of use, but also in the context of the fraction of TST in which obstructive sleep apnea is treated versus untreated or off-PAP sleep time. Quantification of off-PAP sleep time is a potential application of CSTs that would allow us to more precisely demonstrate the true benefits of treating obstructive sleep apnea with CPAP.

Intervention

The continuous, longitudinal monitoring of sleep data with CST devices and management of such data within a patient facing mobile app also confers the opportunity to implement app delivered behavioral sleep interventions that are (1) personalized, given that they are derived with use of the patient's sleep data, (2) dynamic, because interventions can change based on a patient's changing sleep patterns, and (3) real time, because the mobile app delivery of the intervention could be provided near immediately in response to sleep changes. Already, a randomized controlled trial demonstrated benefit of a sleep extension program that integrated a wearable CST and smartphone application. Patients randomized to the technology-assisted program experienced an increase in sleep duration and decrease in sleep disturbances, sleep-related impairments, and blood pressure.[32] Additionally, digital cognitive behavioral therapy for insomnia mobile apps allow for wearable CST-derived sleep parameters to guide therapy.[79,80]

Prediction

Importantly, patterns in the data derived from CSTs may have precision medicine applications outside of sleep disorders, given other illnesses are associated with changes in sleep. For example, analysis of data from 47,249 FitBit users revealed that the incorporation of elevated resting heart rate and increased sleep duration significantly improved predictive models for influenza-like illness.[81] Although these findings were at a state level, with better characterization of sleep patterns associated with different illnesses, data from a CST could alert the patient and their clinician to impending health events. With the recent availability of pulse oximetry readings from CST, predictive capabilities may include exacerbations of congestive heart failure or chronic obstructive pulmonary disease.

From a population health perspective, a U-shaped relationship between sleep duration and the risk of various diseases is well-recognized,[82] and emerging evidence has demonstrated the importance of stability in sleep timing and quality for health.[83] Therefore, CST also holds promise as a tool to further population sleep health; however, a discussion of use cases in detail here is beyond the scope of this article.

Integration with other digital health products

Individuals who use wearable CSTs to track sleep are also likely to harness the other capabilities offered by these devices, such as activity tracking and cardiac arrhythmia identification.[10] Patients may also use other consumer-geared products to quantify additional health metrics simultaneously; for example, mobile apps provide endless opportunities to track caloric intake, alcohol consumption, exercise, menstrual cycles, and mood.[84–86] Additionally, patients may own scales, blood pressure cuffs, pulse oximeters, or other smart devices with wireless connectivity.[84–86]

The continuous glucose monitor (CGM) is a digital health product exemplary of the ability to bridge the gap between consumer-facing tools and medical devices and also demonstrates the usefulness of integrating various sources of health data from mobile technology. Initially, CGM devices for personal use were considered only as an adjunct to traditional glucose readings from finger stick blood samples; however, with improved accuracy, CGM devices are now considered valid for standalone glucose measurement.[87] The mobile apps associated with CGM allow the user (or parent in the pediatric setting) to view real-time blood glucose data, but have evolved over time to improve diabetes self-management.[87] Recently, the FDA cleared a mobile app that aggregates CGM readings, historical insulin dosing, food intake, and physical activity data into an artificial intelligence–based decision support tool to guide insulin dosing and other intervention.[88]

Because sleep impacts numerous health conditions, monitoring sleep data alongside other health parameters in the ambulatory environment could reveal important relationships that guide the development of new interventions. Additionally, new features of wearable technology, such as fall detection by smart watches and physical and social activity tracking through hearing aids, are expected to engage older members of society. Therefore, the sleep field has ample opportunities to understand the role of sleep in health and disease throughout the lifespan.

INTEGRATION INTO TELEMEDICINE AND FUTURE DIRECTIONS

CSTs, whether used for the novel applications described in this article or to substitute traditional actigraphy, could fit seamlessly into a telemedicine program. The ownership of CST by the patient, as opposed the provider, allows for tracking of sleep patterns before a virtual sleep medicine visit. Therefore, instead of retrospective estimates of sleep parameters by the patient at the point of care, a CST deemed acceptable for clinical use would allow the sleep provider to view weeks of sleep patterns before or during the first visit without an in-person exchange. This adjunct information could inform medical decision making during the initial encounter. Because clinical-grade actigraphy devices are unlikely to be provided to patients in advance of the initial visit, this workflow may decrease the time to diagnosis of many non–sleep-disordered breathing conditions that require longitudinal sleep monitoring to satisfy diagnostic criteria.[7] Just like an obstetrics patient presents for a new patient appointment with known results of a commercial pregnancy test, CSTs could provide preliminary information to assist, but never substitute, the comprehensive evaluation and management by an expert clinician.

Additionally, the longitudinal acquisition of objective and subjective patient-generated data by CSTs could be leveraged in an asynchronous store-and-forward telehealth system to hasten the evaluation and treatment of suspected sleep disorders when a sleep provider is not available locally. The sleep specialist might review a collection of electronic health record information (demographics, comorbidities, medications) and patient-generated data derived from a CST (objectively tracked sleep parameters, respiratory information, self-report digital questionnaires, and even oropharyngeal imagery from the smartphone camera). Based on this information, recommendations regarding evaluation and treatment could be provided to the primary care physician.

CSTs may assist with monitoring and interventions between telemedicine visits. As discussed elsewhere in this article, CSTs have been used in conjunction with a cognitive behavioral therapy for insomnia mobile app[79,80] and successfully integrated into a sleep extension protocol[32] that also included coaching through telephone sessions. Innovative methods that use CSTs alongside behavioral therapy are highly complementary to care delivered via telemedicine and can be used when access to behavioral sleep medicine providers is limited. Independent from formal behavioral therapies, between-visit sleep tracking with CSTs may allow patients to visualize improvement in sleep and motivate continued behavioral change and adherence to CPAP or other therapies. Conversely, deterioration in CST-derived sleep parameters, particularly when combined with worsened subjective symptoms, might indicate a need for a change in therapy (eg, adjustment of CPAP settings).

SUMMARY

The opportunities for CSTs to improve sleep health and streamline the telemedicine care of patients with sleep disorders are clear; however, the greatest barrier that impedes adoption by clinicians and researchers is the continued uncertainty that surrounds the ability of CSTs to accurately estimate sleep. Peer-reviewed publications that summarize the performance of currently available CSTs compared with PSG remain limited. Of note, when the performance of a CST is disseminated in the medical and scientific literature, given the proprietary nature of sleep estimation methods, the cited performance values are specific to the device model and firmware, and the associated mobile app software version. Additionally, accuracy cannot be extrapolated beyond the population included in the specific study. Unfortunately, new device models and updated firmware and software iterations are often already in use by the time validation study findings are published, and companies that produce devices with verified performance may go out of business.[58,89–92]

Overcoming the barriers that prevent efficient validation of CSTs will require a collaborative effort between manufacturers, researchers and clinicians. Large datasets composed of raw signal from CSTs co-recorded with PSG in heterogeneous patient populations would create the opportunity for crowdsourcing algorithm training and testing among researchers worldwide.[93] With appropriate disclosure of characteristics of the dataset, open-source code, and performance reporting, researchers could build a library of algorithms appropriate for use in different patient groups. This methodology, which requires a culture of data sharing and significant infrastructure development, would allow for the continued use of available resources while promoting innovation at the level of algorithm development. If minimal technical specifications were delineated for CST housed sensors deemed appropriate for clinical use, such sleep estimation algorithms might be considered device agnostic. An expedited approval method, similar to the FDA precertification program for SaMD, could hasten integration into the health marketplace. However, at this time, validation of CSTs continues in silos and therefore, ambulatory sleep tracking with CSTs has not been standardized for research and clinical practice.

Even if clinicians had greater confidence in the performance of CSTs, systematic integration into clinical sleep medicine is not without pitfalls. Patients may rely more on CST output than their own subjective experience of sleep and, therefore, fail to seek care for underlying sleep disorders. Or, conversely, they may seek care unnecessarily or experience excessive anxiety[94] owing to CST-reported sleep disturbances of unclear clinical significance. Physicians are not immune from an over-reliance on measures from CSTs and may discount patient symptoms that require testing or embark on diagnostic workups in patients without a clear clinical presentation. Additionally, the use of CSTs may increase bias in sleep medicine. Because modern CSTs use machine learning algorithms, which by definition learn from the data provided, individuals with access to CSTs and subspecialty sleep care are overrepresented during algorithm development and CSTs could be less accurate when used in individuals from disadvantaged socioeconomic groups or underserved areas. Other ethical issues might emerge such as breaches to data security and privacy, and CST data could be used to determine employability or culpability in accidents.

Additionally, the collection, transmission, and storage of data from CSTs does not equate to review by a trained health care professional. Cloud-based data from positive airway pressure devices has already required sleep medicine clinics to create workflows for appropriate data management. Similarly, if CSTs are integrated into clinical practice, innovative solutions from the sleep disorders care team will be required to manage the massive influx of patient-generated data from CSTs.

FUNDING

The author's research discussed in this review was supported by the Exercise & Sport Science Initiative University of Michigan; Mobile sleep and circadian rhythm assessment for enhanced athletic performance (U056400).

REFERENCES

1. World market for wearable devices, set to reach $62.82 billion by 2025 - increasing penetration of IoT & related devices drives market growth. Available at: https://www.prnewswire.com/news-releases/world-market-for-wearable-devices-set-to-reach-62-82-billion-by-2025—increasing-penetration-of-iot–related-devices-drives-market-growth-300974593.html. Accessed February 25, 2020.
2. Robbins R, Krebs P, Rapoport DM, et al. Examining use of mobile phones for sleep tracking among a

National sample in the USA. Health Commun 2019; 34:545–51.

3. Berry R, Quan SF, Abreu AR, et al. The AASM manual for the scoring of sleep and associated events: rules, terminology and technical specifications. Version 2.6. Darien, (IL): American Academy of Sleep Medicine; 2020.

4. Ancoli-Israel S, Cole R, Alessi C, et al. The role of actigraphy in the study of sleep and circadian rhythms. Sleep 2003;26:342–92.

5. Sadeh A. The role and validity of actigraphy in sleep medicine: an update. Sleep Med Rev 2011;15: 259–67.

6. Van de Water ATM, Holmes A, Hurley DA. Objective measurements of sleep for non-laboratory settings as alternatives to polysomnography–a systematic review. J Sleep Res 2011;20:183–200.

7. American Academy of Sleep Medicine. International classification of sleep disorders. Darien, (IL): American Academy of Sleep Medicine; 2014.

8. Smith MT, McCrae CS, Cheung J, et al. Use of actigraphy for the evaluation of sleep disorders and circadian rhythm sleep-wake disorders: an American Academy of Sleep Medicine clinical practice guideline. J Clin Sleep Med 2018;14:1231–7.

9. Bianchi MT, Thomas RJ, Westover MB. An open request to epidemiologists: please stop querying self-reported sleep duration. Sleep Med 2017;35: 92–3.

10. Tison GH, Sanchez JM, Ballinger B, et al. Passive detection of atrial fibrillation using a commercially available smartwatch. JAMA Cardiol 2018;3:409–16.

11. de Zambotti M, Cellini N, Menghini L, et al. Sensors capabilities, performance, and use of consumer sleep technology. Sleep Med Clin 2020;15:1–30.

12. Chen KY, Bassett DR. The technology of accelerometry-based activity monitors: current and future. Med Sci Sports Exerc 2005;37:S490–500.

13. Troiano RP, McClain JJ, Brychta RJ, et al. Evolution of accelerometer methods for physical activity research. Br J Sports Med 2014;48:1019–23.

14. Castaneda D, Esparza A, Ghamari M, et al. A review on wearable photoplethysmography sensors and their potential future applications in health care. Int J Biosens Bioelectron 2018;4:195–202.

15. Pereira T, Tran N, Gadhoumi K, et al. Photoplethysmography based atrial fibrillation detection: a review. NPJ Digit Med 2020;3:1–12.

16. US Food and Drug Administration. DEN180042.pdf. Available at: https://www.accessdata.fda.gov/cdrh_docs/reviews/DEN180042.pdf. Accessed February 25, 2020.

17. Charlton PH, Bonnici T, Tarassenko L, et al. An assessment of algorithms to estimate respiratory rate from the electrocardiogram and photoplethysmogram. Physiol Meas 2016;37:610–26.

18. Allen J. Photoplethysmography and its application in clinical physiological measurement. Physiol Meas 2007;28:R1–39.

19. Rayome AD. Fitbit's blood oxygen monitoring feature is here, but what about Apple Watch? CNET. Available at: https://www.cnet.com/news/fitbit-blood-oxygen-monitoring-feature-is-here-but-what-about-apple-watch/. Accessed February 25, 2020.

20. de Zambotti M, Rosas L, Colrain IM, et al. The sleep of the ring: comparison of the ŌURA sleep tracker against polysomnography. Behav Sleep Med 2017; 1–15. https://doi.org/10.1080/15402002.2017. 1300587.

21. Harris J, Lack L, Kemp K, et al. A randomized controlled trial of intensive sleep retraining (ISR): a brief conditioning treatment for chronic insomnia. Sleep 2012;35:49–60.

22. Bianchi MT. Sleep devices: wearables and nearables, informational and interventional, consumer and clinical. Metabolism 2018;84:99–108.

23. Debellemaniere E, Chambon S, Pinaud C, et al. Performance of an ambulatory dry-EEG device for auditory closed-loop stimulation of sleep slow oscillations in the home environment. Front Hum Neurosci 2018;12:88.

24. Schade MM, Bauer CE, Murray BR, et al. Sleep validity of a non-contact bedside movement and respiration-sensing device. J Clin Sleep Med 2019; 15:1051–61.

25. De Chazal P, Fox N, O'HARE EM, et al. Sleep/wake measurement using a non-contact biomotion sensor. J Sleep Res 2011;20:356–66.

26. O'Hare E, Flanagan D, Penzel T, et al. A comparison of radio-frequency biomotion sensors and actigraphy versus polysomnography for the assessment of sleep in normal subjects. Sleep Breath 2015;19: 91–8.

27. Alihanka J, Vaahtoranta K, Saarikivi I. A new method for long-term monitoring of the ballistocardiogram, heart rate, and respiration. Am J Physiol Regul Integr Comp Physiol 1981;240:R384–92.

28. Tuominen J, Peltola K, Saaresranta T, et al. Sleep parameter assessment accuracy of a consumer home sleep monitoring Ballistocardiograph beddit sleep tracker: a validation study. J Clin Sleep Med 2019;15:483–7.

29. Choi YK, Demiris G, Lin SY, et al. Smartphone applications to support sleep self-management: review and evaluation. J Clin Sleep Med 2018;14:1783–90.

30. Fino E, Mazzetti M. Monitoring healthy and disturbed sleep through smartphone applications: a review of experimental evidence. Sleep Breath 2019;23: 13–24.

31. Borger JN, Huber R, Ghosh A. Capturing sleep–wake cycles by using day-to-day smartphone touchscreen interactions. NPJ Digit Med 2019;2:1–8.

32. Baron KG, Duffecy J, Richardson D, et al. Technology assisted behavior intervention to extend sleep among adults with short sleep duration and prehypertension/stage 1 hypertension: a randomized pilot feasibility study. J Clin Sleep Med 2019;15:1587–97.

33. Kushida CA, Chang A, Gadkary C, et al. Comparison of actigraphic, polysomnographic, and subjective assessment of sleep parameters in sleep-disordered patients. Sleep Med 2001;2:389–96.

34. Sadeh A, Sharkey KM, Carskadon MA. Activity-based sleep-wake identification: an empirical test of methodological issues. Sleep 1994;17:201–7.

35. Cole RJ, Kripke DF, Gruen W, et al. Automatic sleep/wake identification from wrist activity. Sleep 1992;15:461–9.

36. Natale V, Drejak M, Erbacci A, et al. Monitoring sleep with a smartphone accelerometer. Sleep Biol Rhythms 2012;10:287–92.

37. Beattie Z, Oyang Y, Statan A, et al. Estimation of sleep stages in a healthy adult population from optical plethysmography and accelerometer signals. Physiol Meas 2017;38:1968–79.

38. Zhang X, Kou W, Eric I, et al. Sleep stage classification based on multi-level feature learning and recurrent neural networks via wearable device. Comput Biol Med 2018;103:71–81.

39. Walch O, Huang Y, Forger D, et al. Sleep stage prediction with raw acceleration and photoplethysmography heart rate data derived from a consumer wearable device. Sleep 2019;42.

40. Fonseca P, Weysen T, Goelema MS, et al. Validation of photoplethysmography-based sleep staging compared with polysomnography in healthy middle-aged adults. Sleep 2017;40(7).

41. van Hees VT, Sabia S, Jones SE. Estimating sleep parameters using an accelerometer without sleep diary. Sci Rep 2018;8:1–11.

42. Younes M, Raneri J, Hanly P. Staging sleep in polysomnograms: analysis of inter-scorer variability. J Clin Sleep Med 2016;12:885–94.

43. Danker-Hopfe H, Anderer P, Zeitlhofer J, et al. Inter-rater reliability for sleep scoring according to the Rechtschaffen & Kales and the new AASM standard. J Sleep Res 2009;18:74–84.

44. Depner CM, Cheng PC, Devine JK, et al. Wearable technologies for developing sleep and circadian biomarkers: a summary of workshop discussions. Sleep 2020;43:zsz254.

45. de Zambotti M, Cellini N, Goldstone A, et al. Wearable sleep technology in clinical and research settings. Med Sci Sports Exerc 2019;51:1538–57.

46. Toon E, Davey MJ, Hollis SL, et al. Comparison of commercial wrist-based and smartphone accelerometers, actigraphy, and PSG in a clinical cohort of children and adolescents. J Clin Sleep Med 2016;12:343–50.

47. Pesonen A-K, Kuula L. The validity of a new consumer-targeted wrist device in sleep measurement: an overnight comparison against polysomnography in children and adolescents. J Clin Sleep Med 2018;14:585–91.

48. Lee XK, Chee NI, Ong JL, et al. Validation of a consumer sleep wearable device with actigraphy and polysomnography in adolescents across sleep opportunity manipulations. J Clin Sleep Med 2019;15:1337–46.

49. Tonetti L, Cellini N, de Zambotti M, et al. Polysomnographic validation of a wireless dry headband technology for sleep monitoring in healthy young adults. Physiol Behav 2013;118:185–8.

50. Shambroom JR, Fábregas SE, Johnstone J. Validation of an automated wireless system to monitor sleep in healthy adults. J Sleep Res 2012;21:221–30.

51. Tal A, Shinar Z, Shaki D, et al. Validation of contact-free sleep monitoring device with comparison to polysomnography. J Clin Sleep Med 2017;13:517–22.

52. Bhat S, Ferraris A, Gupta D, et al. Is there a clinical role for smartphone sleep apps? Comparison of sleep cycle detection by a smartphone application to polysomnography. J Clin Sleep Med 2015;11:709–15.

53. Patel P, Kim JY, Brooks LJ. Accuracy of a smartphone application in estimating sleep in children. Sleep Breath 2017;21:505–11.

54. de Zambotti M, Baker FC, Willoughby AR, et al. Measures of sleep and cardiac functioning during sleep using a multi-sensory commercially-available wristband in adolescents. Physiol Behav 2016;158:143–9.

55. Haghayegh S, Khoshnevis S, Smolensky MH, et al. Accuracy of PurePulse photoplethysmography technology of Fitbit Charge 2 for assessment of heart rate during sleep. Chronobiol Int 2019;36:927–33.

56. de Zambotti M, Goldstone A, Claudatos S, et al. A validation study of Fitbit Charge 2™ compared with polysomnography in adults. Chronobiol Int 2018;35:465–76.

57. Cook JD, Eftekari SC, Dallmann E, et al. Ability of the Fitbit Alta HR to quantify and classify sleep in patients with suspected central disorders of hypersomnolence: a comparison against polysomnography. J Sleep Res 2019;28:e12789.

58. Cook JD, Prairie ML, Plante DT. Ability of the multi-sensory Jawbone UP3 to quantify and classify sleep in patients with suspected central disorders of hypersomnolence: a comparison against polysomnography and actigraphy. J Clin Sleep Med 2018;14:841–8.

59. Sargent C, Lastella M, Romyn G, et al. How well does a commercially available wearable device

measure sleep in young athletes? Chronobiol Int 2018;35:754–8.

60. Kang SG, Kang JM, Ko KP, et al. Validity of a commercial wearable sleep tracker in adult insomnia disorder patients and good sleepers. J Psychosom Res 2017; 97:38–44.

61. Meltzer LJ, Hiruma LS, Avis K, et al. Comparison of a commercial accelerometer with polysomnography and actigraphy in children and adolescents. Sleep 2015;38:1323–30.

62. Gruwez A, Bruyneel A-V, Bruyneel M. The validity of two commercially-available sleep trackers and actigraphy for assessment of sleep parameters in obstructive sleep apnea patients. PLoS One 2019; 14:e0210569.

63. Moreno-Pino F, Porras-Segovia A, López-Esteban P, et al. Validation of fitbit charge 2 and fitbit alta HR against polysomnography for assessing sleep in adults with obstructive sleep apnea. J Clin Sleep Med 2019;15:1645–53.

64. Guber A, Epstein Shochet G, Kohn S, et al. Wrist-sensor pulse oximeter enables prolonged patient monitoring in chronic lung diseases. J Med Syst 2019;43:230.

65. Berryhill S, Morton CJ, Dean A, et al. Effect of wearables on sleep in healthy individuals: a randomized cross-over trial and validation study. J Clin Sleep Med 2020;16(5):775–83.

66. Huysmans D, Borzée P, Testelmans D, et al. Evaluation of a commercial ballistocardiography sensor for sleep apnea screening and sleep monitoring. Sensors 2019;19 [pii:E2133].

67. Agatsuma T, Fujimoto K, Komatsu Y, et al. A novel device (SD-101) with high accuracy for screening sleep apnoea-hypopnoea syndrome. Respirology 2009;14:1143–50.

68. Norman MB, Middleton S, Erskine O, et al. Validation of the Sonomat: a contactless monitoring system used for the diagnosis of sleep disordered breathing. Sleep 2014;37:1477–87.

69. Zaffaroni A, Kent B, O'Hare E, et al. Assessment of sleep-disordered breathing using a non-contact bio-motion sensor. J Sleep Res 2013;22:231–6.

70. Behar J, Roebuck A, Shahid M, et al. SleepAp: an automated obstructive sleep apnoea screening application for smartphones. IEEE J Biomed Health Inform 2015;19:325–31.

71. Nakano H, Hirayama K, Sadamitsu Y, et al. Monitoring sound to quantify snoring and sleep apnea severity using a smartphone: proof of concept. J Clin Sleep Med 2014;10:73–8.

72. Khosla S, Deak MC, Gault D, et al. Consumer sleep technology: an American Academy of sleep medicine position statement. J Clin Sleep Med 2018;14:877–80.

73. US Food and Drug Administration. Digital health software precertification (Pre-Cert) program. 2019. Available at: https://www.fda.gov/medical-devices/digital-health/digital-health-software-precertification-pre-cert-program. Accessed February 25, 2020.

74. Gonçalves BSB, Adamowicz T, Louzada FM, et al. A fresh look at the use of nonparametric analysis in actimetry. Sleep Med Rev 2015;20:84–91.

75. Fossion R, Rivera AL, Toledo-Roy JC, et al. Multi-scale adaptive analysis of circadian rhythms and intradaily variability: application to actigraphy time series in acute insomnia subjects. PLoS One 2017; 12:e0181762.

76. McEvoy RD, Antic NA, Heeley E, et al. CPAP for prevention of cardiovascular events in obstructive sleep apnea. N Engl J Med 2016;375:919–31.

77. da Silva Paulitsch F, Zhang L. Continuous positive airway pressure for adults with obstructive sleep apnea and cardiovascular disease: a meta-analysis of randomized trials. Sleep Med 2019;54:28–34.

78. Thomas RJ, Bianchi MT. Urgent need to improve PAP management: the devil is in two (fixable) details. J Clin Sleep Med 2017;13:657–64.

79. Kang SG, Kang JM, Cho SJ, et al. Cognitive behavioral therapy using a mobile application synchronizable with wearable devices for insomnia treatment: a pilot study. J Clin Sleep Med 2017;13:633–40.

80. Luik AI, Farias Machado P, Espie CA. Delivering digital cognitive behavioral therapy for insomnia at scale: does using a wearable device to estimate sleep influence therapy? NPJ Digit Med 2018;1:3.

81. Radin JM, Wineinger NE, Topol EJ, et al. Harnessing wearable device data to improve state-level real-time surveillance of influenza-like illness in the USA: a population-based study. Lancet Digit Health 2020;2:e85–93.

82. Consensus Conference Panel, Watson NF, Badr MS, et al. Joint consensus statement of the American Academy of Sleep Medicine and Sleep Research Society on the recommended amount of sleep for a healthy adult: methodology and discussion. Sleep 2015;38:1161–83.

83. Bei B, Wiley JF, Trinder J, et al. Beyond the mean: a systematic review on the correlates of daily intraindividual variability of sleep/wake patterns. Sleep Med Rev 2016;28:108–24.

84. Jain SH, Powers BW, Hawkins JB, et al. The digital phenotype. Nat Biotechnol 2015;33:462–3.

85. Steinhubl SR, Muse ED, Topol EJ. The emerging field of mobile health. Sci Transl Med 2015;7:283rv3.

86. Topol EJ. A decade of digital medicine innovation. Sci Transl Med 2019;11 [pii:eaaw7610].

87. Battelino T, Danne T, Bergenstal RM, et al. Clinical targets for continuous glucose monitoring data interpretation: recommendations from the international consensus on time in range. Diabetes Care 2019; 42:1593–603.

88. DreaMed advisor - turning patient data into treatment insight. DreaMed. Available at: https://

dreamed-diabetes.com/advisor/. Accessed February 25, 2020.

89. Griessenberger H, Heib DPJ, Kunz AB, et al. Assessment of a wireless headband for automatic sleep scoring. Sleep Breath 2013;17:747–52.

90. de Zambotti M, Baker FC, Colrain IM. Validation of sleep-tracking technology compared with polysomnography in adolescents. Sleep 2015;38:1461–8.

91. Sleep tracking startup Zeo says goodnight. TechCrunch. Available at: https://social.techcrunch.com/2013/05/22/sleep-tracking-startup-zeo-says-goodnight/. Accessed February 25, 2020.

92. Failed startups: Jawbone. Available at: https://www.forbes.com/sites/maryjuetten/2019/02/05/failed-startups-jawbone/#66235b775b6d. Accessed February 25, 2020.

93. van Gilst MM, van Dijk JP, Krijn R, et al. Protocol of the SOMNIA project: an observational study to create a neurophysiological database for advanced clinical sleep monitoring. BMJ Open 2019;9: e030996.

94. Baron KG, Abbott S, Jao N, et al. Orthosomnia: are some patients taking the quantified self too far? J Clin Sleep Med 2017;13:351–4.

Regulatory, Legal, and Ethical Considerations of Telemedicine

Barry G. Fields, MD, MSEd*

KEYWORDS

- Telemedicine • Interstate licensure compact • Informed consent • Stark law • Ryan Haight act
- Protected health information

KEY POINTS

- Telemedicine practitioners should follow applicable practice regulations at the facility, state, and federal levels.
- Streamlined multistate medical licensing now exists through the Interstate Medical Licensure Compact.
- Practitioners should collaborate with their malpractice insurers to ensure appropriate coverage.
- The same ethical, conflict of interest, and personal health information protection obligations exist for practicing telemedicine as practicing in-person medicine.

INTRODUCTION

Telemedicine has been regulated almost as long as it has existed. Five states had adopted legislation by 1992, a number that grew to 15 states within 3 years. A quarter of a century later, all 50 states now have laws pertaining to telemedicine.[1] Federal statutes and any facility-based regulations are superimposed on that state-based legislation, resulting in a tangle of rules than can frustrate even the most committed sleep telemedicine practitioner.

The purpose of this article is not to stymie the field with lists of regulations, laws, and ethical dilemmas. On the contrary, it is meant to guide telemedicine practitioners and other stakeholders (heath system administrators, practice managers, and so forth) through the broad brushstrokes of these topics while identifying useful resources for more in-depth study (**Box 1**). Even if this article does not provide answers to every applicable question, it should aid these individuals in learning which questions to ask.

Much of the article can be summarized in 3 words: know your state. Or, more precisely,

know your state's rules (distant site) and the rules pertaining to the states in which your patients reside (originating sites). States have instituted different regulations regarding practices before, during, and after clinic encounters. For instance, some states require patients to complete a written informed consent form before telemedicine visits can begin. Others require an in-person visit be performed before engaging in telemedicine-based follow-up. Learning these details about the states in which care is provided is essential; disobeying telemedicine regulations can have professional and legal consequence for both providers and their workplaces, as the following case study illustrates.

A CASE STUDY: HAGESETH V. SUPERIOR COURT

In 2005, a California resident attempted to purchase fluoxetine online for his ongoing moderate depression. The Web site operators, based outside the United States, forwarded his request and associated questionnaires to Colorado

Department of Pulmonary, Allergy, Critical Care, and Sleep Medicine, Emory University School of Medicine, Atlanta VA Health Care System, Atlanta, GA, USA
* Atlanta VA Sleep Medicine Center, 250 North Arcadia Avenue, Decatur, GA 30030.
E-mail address: barry.fields@emory.edu

Sleep Med Clin 15 (2020) 409–416
https://doi.org/10.1016/j.jsmc.2020.06.004
1556-407X/20/Published by Elsevier Inc.

Box 1
Major legal and regulatory considerations

- Informed consent
- Licensing
- Clinical privileges and credentials
- Internet prescribing
- Conflicts of interest
- Malpractice insurance
- Protected health information

---

psychiatrist Dr Christian Hageseth. Dr Hageseth neither conducted a face-to-face evaluation of the patient nor was licensed to practice medicine in California. After reviewing the questionnaire information, Dr Hageseth issued an online prescription for the medication. A Mississippi pharmacy filled the prescription and sent it to the patient. Several weeks later, the patient completed suicide. Postmortem bloodwork revealed detectable fluoxetine levels. The San Mateo County District Attorney charged Dr Hageseth with practicing medicine in California without a license. He challenged the charges, claiming that the court lacked jurisdiction because his prescribing behavior took place outside of California. However, the California Court of Appeals ruled against this challenge and Dr Hageseth pled guilty. He was sentenced to 9 months in prison.[2]

Although *Hageseth v. Superior Court* involves a particular form of telemedicine (Internet-based prescribing), it raises many questions that are applicable to other forms of telemedicine as well:

1. Should a patient provide informed consent before beginning telemedicine-based treatment, absolving the prescriber of all or most potential harms that could arise?
2. Can a provider licensed in one state treat a patient located in another state?
3. Are providers allowed to order medication over the Internet (controlled substance or not) for patients they have never evaluated beyond questionnaires?
4. Must providers have the same privileges at a health care facility–based originating site as they would if physically providing care there?
5. What conflict of interest regulations apply?
6. Does medical malpractice insurance cover telemedicine?
7. What personal health information (PHI) regulations should be considered?

Each of these topics is reviewed here, followed by a discussion of ethical standards as they pertain to sleep telemedicine, such as: what are the ethical duties of prescribers who have never physically met, or even interacted, with their patients?

INFORMED CONSENT

Informed consent requirements vary by state; there is no federal policy. Some states require a written acknowledgment form completed and signed by the patient, whereas other states have no such requirements. As noted in the Ethics section later, informed consent is an important part of telemedicine initiation whether documentation to that effect is required or not. The Federation of State Medical Boards (FSMB) suggests the following elements be included in informed consent:[3]

- Documentation of the patient, provider, and credentials
- Type of telemedicine being used (face to face, online prescribing, and so forth)
- Recognition that the practitioner may decide whether managing a particular condition is appropriate via telemedicine
- Security measures taken to protect PHI, and potential privacy risks
- Clause holding providers harmless for information loss caused by technical failure
- Requirement for patient consent to forward PHI to a third party

Of course, these are only suggestions for states and their providers. Individual telemedicine practitioners may wish to develop their own informed consent forms in conjunction with legal counsel not only to enhance patient disclosure processes but also to reduce potential legal exposure should negative outcomes arise. *Hageseth v. Superior Court* reveals a potential vulnerability when no such documentation of risk acknowledgment exists. Among other deficiencies, Dr Hageseth had no record of patient consent to his method of care.

LICENSING

In general, practitioners must be licensed in the states in which their originating site patients reside. Licensing requirements vary significantly by state; knowing both originating state and distant state rules before implementing a telemedicine program is essential. Detailed information is available through the National Telehealth Policy Resource Center, a component of the Center for Connected Health Policy (CCHP): https://www.cchpca.org/about/projects/national-telehealth-policy-resource-center.

The CCHP notes that 9 states issue special licenses or certificates allowing out-of-state licensed practitioners to practice telemedicine with patients in their states: Alabama, Louisiana, Maine, Minnesota, New Mexico, Ohio, Oregon, Tennessee, and Texas. State-specific rules apply regarding what constitutes telemedicine, and whether these practitioners are then prohibited from opening brick-and-mortar practices in the state.[2]

Federal legislation easing interstate licensing restrictions has slowly materialized with the advent of the Interstate Medical Licensure Compact (IMLC), developed by FSMB. Twenty-nine states, the District of Columbia, and Guam are now part of the IMLC, with more states joining annually. Although a license obtained through the IMLC costs physicians more than licenses obtained conventionally (standard state licensing fee plus FSMB fee), significant time and effort is saved because a single online application may be used to apply for licensure in multiple states. There are specific physician qualifications to participate, including maintaining unrestricted licensure in the state of principle licensure, remaining board certified in the specialty of practice, and having no history of disciplinary actions against the license. The FSMB outlines additional qualifications on their Web site: www.fsmb.org. Consulting the IMLC Web site in the context of our case study shows that Dr Hageseth would still be prohibited from treating California patients through telemedicine unless he obtained a California medical license through traditional methods; although Colorado is part of the IMLC, California is not.

Like many other specialties, sleep medicine is becoming more focused on a team-based model of care.[4] Therefore, licensing concerns are not only limited to physicians and advanced care providers (ACPs; physician assistants and nurse practitioners) but also to nurses and polysomnogram (PSG) technicians. Nurses must hold licenses in both the state in which they reside and the state in which the patient is located. Similar to the IMLC, a nursing licensure compact now exists among 25 states. Interstate PSG technician licensing is more variable; individual state policy should be consulted. For instance, some medical boards (eg, Idaho, Tennessee, New York, and California) have specific technician licensing requirements.[5] In addition, nurses and technicians must consider scope of practice when conducting telemedicine visits. Like ACPs, their allowable scope can differ among states. In sum, sleep nurses and technicians should ensure that they are both (1) licensed in the state where the patient is located (if applicable for technicians) and (2) practicing within the scope of practice regulations in that state. In another nuance, nurses may only take orders from physicians or ACPs licensed in the patient's state; orders from providers unlicensed in that state are invalid.[6]

CLINICAL PRIVILEGES AND CREDENTIALS

Like traditional care providers, telemedicine providers must obtain treatment privileges and be credentialed at any health care facility in which they practice. This requirement can lead to substantial administrative burden on both the provider and the facility. However, facilitated processes do exist for federally defined Critical Access Hospitals. Congress created this designation in 1997 in response to many rural hospitals closing in the late 1980s and early 1990s. Therefore, part of the federal government's goal is to stabilize the number of practitioners available to provide care within them; telemedicine-based care is a vital part of this strategy. In 2011, Centers for Medicare and Medicaid Services (CMS) decreased the burden on both distant-site providers and Critical Access Hospitals (originating sites) by allowing providers' distant-site credentials to be accepted at originating sites. This credentialing by proxy option is available to hospitals meeting specific criteria:[7]

- Written agreement between originating and distant site
- Distant site is a Medicare-participating hospital or telemedicine entity
- Telemedicine provider is privileged at distant-site hospital, with those privileges provided to originating site
- Telemedicine provider holds a license in originating site's state
- Originating site hospital reviews provider's performance and provides this information to distant-site hospital
- Originating site hospital informs distant-site hospital of all adverse events and complaints related to the telemedicine provider

Therefore, sleep providers wishing to conduct telemedicine visits to a Critical Access Hospital need not repeat the credentialing process at that facility as long as they have completed it at a distant site. If that Critical Access Hospital is located in a state in which the provider is licensed, the process (from a legal and regulatory standpoint) is even more straightforward.

INTERNET PRESCRIBING

As telemedicine has grown, so have concerns about practitioners' prescribing controlled substances for patients whom they have never physically seen or examined. States vary in their

Internet-based prescribing regulations, especially when the prescriber resides out of state. Any policies from both the medical and pharmacy boards should be reviewed before implementing a telemedicine program in any state in which the care occurs.

Like several areas discussed, federal law overlays state policy. The Ryan Haight Online Pharmacy Consumer Protection Act of 2008 regulates this area. The act, designed to prevent illegal distribution and dispensing of controlled substances via the Internet, added new provisions to the already-established Controlled Substances Act. Its overall message is that no controlled substance "may be delivered, distributed, or dispensed by means of the Internet without a valid prescription."[8] A key part of the "valid prescription" definition is that the prescriber, or a covering prescriber, must perform at least 1 in-person medical evaluation of the patient.[8]

Although the act recognizes the practice of telemedicine as an exception to this rule, it stops short of delineating a special registration pathway that would allow telemedicine practitioners to prescribe through the Internet without in-person evaluation. The act states: "The Attorney General may issue to a practitioner a special registration to engage in the practice of telemedicine."[8] Although this special registration process was never enacted, changes are afoot. Substance Use-Disorder Prevention that Promotes Opiate Recover and Treatment (SUPPORT) for Patients and Communities Act of 2018 set a 10/24/19 deadline for the Attorney General to activate that provision.

As of this writing, there is no finalized, public guidance in response to that deadline. However, it is anticipated that telemedicine practitioners will soon learn of a specific registration process that will allow them to comply with Drug Enforcement Agency (DEA) regulations and the Ryan Haight Act while still performing telemedicine without in-person examination requirements.

CONFLICTS OF INTEREST

Sleep telemedicine providers must adhere to the same federal standards regarding real or perceived conflicts of interest as they would as in-person sleep medicine providers. These situations include providing or accepting goods or services simply to encourage referrals (anti-kickback laws). For instance, if a distant-site provider purchases telemedicine equipment for a Critical Access Hospital with hopes of establishing it as an originating site, that action could be viewed as a form of inducement. If such behavior results in

remuneration to the offender under a federal health care program, it is an Anti-Kickback Statute–associated felony punishable by steep fines and/or imprisonment.[5]

Another potential conflict of interest occurs when telemedicine providers leverage their programs to increase business traffic to their own business ventures. The federal self-referral law, or Stark Law, applies to every practitioner whether care is provided through telemedicine or in-person methods. For instance, the Stark Law prohibits providers from billing Medicare if selling patients durable medical equipment from a company in which they have a financial stake. Sleep testing is outside of the Stark Law and, therefore, a sleep provider ordering testing in a self-owned sleep laboratory is permissible as long as the laboratory is not performed in a hospital (and, even then, it may be allowed in some situations). Stark Law does not apply if nonfederal reimbursement is sought for goods and services.

In addition to federal rules addressing conflicts of interest, many states possess their own legislation regarding kickbacks, self-referrals, and the like. Sleep telemedicine providers should familiarize themselves with applicable laws at all originating sites; it is these rules against which their conduct will be judged if seeking federally sourced reimbursement.

MALPRACTICE INSURANCE

This topic, more than any other, is most heavily dependent on a practitioner's specific situation. Before implementing any telemedicine program, liability exposure should be mitigated. There are 2 primary questions to consider. Does the malpractice policy cover (1) telemedicine and (2) care provided outside of the states in which the clinician currently practices? Telemedicine-related claim coverage should be stipulated explicitly in the policy documents. Similarly, policies must indicate the jurisdictions in which claims are covered; practitioners may find that although *intrastate* telemedicine may be within their policy's coverage, *interstate* telemedicine is not. These malpractice insurance considerations extend beyond practitioners (physicians, ACPs) to other sleep medicine teammates as well, such as nurses.[6]

PROTECTED HEALTH INFORMATION

Providers' approach to PHI during telemedicine should be the same as it is for in-person visits. Health Insurance Portability and Accountability Act (HIPAA) requirements must be followed in addition to any state, local, or institutional/

organizational standards. Software used should be patched with the latest security updates, and the operating system used should be up to date. Notably, PHI is not limited to medical reports. Patients' email addresses, phone numbers, street addresses, and so forth are all in this category and must all be protected. State privacy laws vary in their stringency depending on the technology used; the National Telehealth Policy Resource Center provides more state-specific information: https://www.cchpca.org/about/projects/national-telehealth-policy-resource-center.

Any communication and data storage systems should be encrypted and password protected, with telemedicine practitioners educated on best practices to protect PHI. Inactivity timeout functionality is recommended. Only authorized users should have access to telemedicine systems, with unauthorized access attempts recorded and reviewable.[9] Collaboration with data security experts/computer technicians is generally recommended. Audio and video recording is discouraged given patient consent considerations and susceptibility to hacking.[6]

Sleep telemedicine is unique in its significant reliance on store-and-forward telemedicine technology in patient assessment and decision making. Protected access to previous sleep testing is often required, with any data from that testing transferred directly into the secure patient records. Providers must use positive airway pressure (PAP) data collection platforms offering cybersecurity protection of patient data on their Web site. These sites are restricted either to a practice group or an individual provider (eg, Airview and EncoreAnywhere).

ETHICS

Like any emerging technology, telemedicine-related hardware and software come with no ethical dilemmas in themselves. It is how this technology is used that can create ethical conundrums. The American Medical Association (AMA) outlines ethical obligations between a patient and provider along a continuum reflecting the type of telemedicine used (levels of accountability).[10] At 1 end of this continuum are Web sites providing only indirect interaction between a patient and provider. Although the medical professional is responsible for the general accuracy of content presented, there is no direct responsibility and little accountability for how readers will use that information. Web sites guiding patients through the steps of insomnia treatment are good examples. Further along the continuum are non–real-time platforms for patients' sleep study data, so-called asynchronous or store-and-forward telemedicine. In this scenario, the distant-site provider is responsible for making an accurate diagnosis that will guide the patient's care. However, it could be another provider who makes treatment decisions based on those findings. Both the interpreting and treating providers share responsibility for keeping with in-person standards (confidentiality, adequate training to perform the task, and so forth).[10]

When telemedicine and treatment initiation are provided by the same person (as in *Hageseth v. Superior Court*), more ethical dilemmas arise. The following ethical discussion focuses on provider-patient interactions at the most interactive end of the telemedicine spectrum: real-time, synchronous, clinical video telehealth (CVT). Four widely accepted principles of medical ethics should be respected in developing and sustaining any sleep CVT program:[11]

1. Autonomy: patients' right to make decisions about their medical care
2. Beneficence: a provider's duty to benefit the patient in all situations
3. Nonmaleficence: a provider's duty to harm neither the patient nor society during the care of that patient
4. Justice: a provider's duty to ensure fairness in medical decisions, implying equal distribution of scarce resources and new treatments, and upholding applicable laws and legislation

Autonomy

If a sleep medicine patient's autonomy in decision making is to be supported, the patient needs as much information as possible about both the care recommended and the manner in which it is provided (ie, telemedicine vs in-person care). Respecting this principle begins when the patient is first referred to the sleep clinic. If both telemedicine and in-person care options exist, and the condition is likely equally well managed through both modalities, then the patient should be made aware of both options. It should not be assumed that a patient would prefer a telemedicine encounter to an in-person evaluation, even if the individual lives far from a sleep center or experiences disability. Conversely, it should not be assumed that a local patient free from disability would be best served by in-person care. In either case, patients should receive information about both treatment formats at the time of scheduling without an opt-in or opt-out bias guiding the discussion. Once both options are fully presented, patients can then make a more informed decision about how they wish to receive their care.

This decision-making process incorporates several assumptions. First, because it is typically scheduling staff who initiate communication with patients, it behooves practitioners and practice managers to ensure these individuals are themselves informed enough about telemedicine to educate patients effectively. Supporting patients' autonomy is heavily dependent on accurate information sharing at this point of initial contact; withholding information either voluntarily or unwittingly undermines these efforts. Second, the decision-making process described assumes that practitioners are just as able to treat one patient through telemedicine as any other. This situation is not always the case. As described in relation to licensing, practitioners may not have the licensing and credentials to treat a patient if the visit originates from another state; legal considerations sometimes preclude patient choice. Third, telemedicine can be difficult to explain over the phone even for the most experienced scheduling personnel and savviest of patients. Nuances, including audio quality, telemedicine presenter interaction, and loss of physical practitioner-patient touch, may not be fully appreciated until the patient arrives for the first telemedicine visit. Autonomy must then be supported if a patient wishes to reverse an earlier decision and pursue in-person care; it should be made explicit to the patient that initiating telemedicine does not preclude future in-person visits.

Respecting patients' autonomy goes beyond choices in health care setting. Sleep telemedicine practitioners must ensure patient privacy to the same extent they would during in-person visits. It should not be assumed that information gleaned from patient encounters (verbal information, sleep testing results, PAP data) may be shared with any other entity unless specified by the patient. Other individuals in the room with the patient at the originating site should be identified, and providers should ask patients explicitly if they will allow others to remain in the room throughout the interview no matter what material is discussed. Similarly, providers at the distant site should identify anyone else in the room with them, including trainees, nurses, or administrative staff. A patient's autonomy is eroded if anyone, on either side of the interaction, has access to the PHI without the patient's knowledge and permission.

Beneficence

Once patients choose to participate in a telemedicine-based treatment pathway, providers and associated personnel must uphold the highest standards of care during their sleep medicine journeys. Part of that obligation comes through education. It is not feasible to assume that clinicians can transition seamlessly from in-person patient care to telemedicine-based care without training, both didactic and experiential. Although multiple specialties have recognized this need and committed themselves to formalizing telemedicine education (dermatology, emergency medicine, neurology), sleep medicine has lagged behind. Recent research shows that most physicians without telemedicine experience are uncomfortable evaluating new patients (75%) and making diagnosis and treatment decisions through telemedicine (95%).[11] However, studies with providers having more telemedicine experience reveal more positive attitudes toward the modality. Providers think that telemedicine's impact on patient-provider interactions is neutral to, or even more positive than, in-person visits.[12,13]

Beyond an initial visit, sleep telemedicine providers should use patient satisfaction and quality improvement monitoring to ensure the principle of beneficence remains upheld. In 2015, the American Academy of Sleep Medicine (AASM) introduced a series of quality measures for adult obstructive sleep apnea (OSA),[14] pediatric OSA,[15] narcolepsy,[16] restless legs syndrome (RLS),[17] and insomnia.[18] Although designed to be measured and tracked in more traditional, in-person environments, every quality measure may also be adapted for the telemedicine clinic. For instance, the same RLS symptom severity questionnaires used in an in-person clinic may also be used for telemedicine; questionnaires can be located at an originating clinic for center-to-center (C2C) telemedicine or emailed to a patient for center-to-home (C2H) telemedicine. The responses can then be transmitted to the distant site using encrypted systems with the patient's permission. In the OSA realm, most PAP machines have wireless data download capability. Treatment adherence and effectiveness can be reviewed via the Internet with a patient using screen-share technology. Therefore, by subtle adaptations to in-person clinic practice, telemedicine in no way precludes practitioners from ensuring beneficence for their patients while meeting AASM quality measure goals.

Nonmaleficence

Although telemedicine has been used to decrease travel burden on patients, the modality can also have unintended negative effects. The principle of nonmaleficence addresses this issue. Fear can be a significant issue among patients and families even if they initially agree to partake in the technology. As alluded to earlier, telemedicine-naive patients may relish the prospect of staying home or close to home for their sleep medicine care. However, considering the full implications of the visit as it draws nearer can be unsettling. Unfamiliar technology coupled with an unknown medical provider far away can prove stressful, even overwhelming.[11] Providers and other staff members should remain sensitive to these concerns and how they evolve over time. Patients may be calmed to learn that telemedicine is simply a tool to provide standard medical care, staff will be available to assist with the technology (especially for C2C visits), and patients may choose to switch to in-person care at any time. These techniques can decrease the unintended burden on patients often already encumbered by other issues and concerns.

In addition to these important but well-intentioned challenges to the principle of nonmaleficence, more malignant threats exist. Telemedicine-associated equipment can be expensive. Therefore, practitioners must use it for many patients to recuperate the cost and obtain a profit. A conflict of interest can then arise when patients who might otherwise have been offered in-person care are scheduled for telemedicine-based care, regardless of their wishes (diminishing their autonomy), medical complexity, and providers' experience with the technology. As one bioethicist wrote, "At that moment the technological imperative transforms the healing profession into a healthcare enterprise and our patients become a means to an end."[11] Nevertheless, the same reimbursement restrictions that have slowed sleep telemedicine's growth have also curbed the potential for its misuse. Because practitioners receive little to no additional reimbursement for telemedicine encounters compared with in-person visits, there is less motivation to choose one modality rather than the other (especially once telemedicine technology costs have been recovered). It is yet to be seen how changes in health care reimbursement as a whole may affect how nonmaleficence is maintained.

Justice

Ideally, every patient should have the same access to telemedicine for part or all of their sleep medicine care. However, the same provider shortages that plague the specialty also apply to telemedicine. The AASM estimates there are only about 7500 board-certified sleep specialists to serve more than 350 million Americans. Therefore, there is 1 sleep specialist for about every 43,000 Americans, with most sleep providers concentrated in states such as New York, Florida, Texas, and California.[4] There are current efforts to widen the training pipeline, but real shortages in terms of provider numbers and geography will persist. It is this area where telemedicine has greatest potential to improve treatment equity and justice.

However, there are significant challenges to consider. Socioeconomically disadvantaged Americans face the same limited access to telemedicine care as they would in-person care. Fiscally responsible telemedicine programs rely on adequate reimbursement to sustain them, typically from public payors, private payors, and out-of-pocket from patients. Uninsured or underinsured Americans often lack each of these sources, perpetuating telemedicine inaccessibility. Another factor affecting justice in telemedicine dissemination is geography. Although one benefit of telemedicine is overcoming geographic challenges, rural patients accessing C2C telemedicine often travel long distances to do so. Difficulties accessing reliable transportation, missed work hours, and variable weather conditions are all potential burdens. Although C2H telemedicine can ameliorate some of these issues, it relies on patients possessing feasible equipment (smartphone, tablet, computer) to make the connection. Furthermore, some payors who cover C2C visits do not reimburse for C2H visits. For instance, as of early 2020, Medicare only covered C2H for specific purposes, which do not include sleep medicine. Long term plans to sustain temporary, Covid-19 related coverage benefits for C2H telemedicine are yet to be determined.

Telemedicine program developers must consider each of these factors in designing programs enhancing justice and access equity among all patients served. The US Department of Veterans' Affairs (VA) system has made progress in this regard. Supported by the VA MISSION Act, computer tablets with webcams can be sent to veterans for variable amounts of time. With those devices, any veteran may choose to participate in C2H using the VA-issued hardware. Use outcomes are being tracked, but preliminary data show significant impact among veterans throughout the nation.[19]

SUMMARY

Navigating the regulatory system underlying sleep telemedicine in 2020 requires preparation, commitment, and attention to detail; however, so does navigating the same system for in-person care. Telemedicine is unique in some ways. Prescribers may need to consider multiple states' regulations, and work through nuances such as multistate licensing and credentialing. In other ways, telemedicine is simply another way to practice medicine. Conflict of interest (real or perceived) should be avoided, PHI should be protected, and the highest of ethical standards should be upheld. With that recognition of more similarity than dissimilarity will come improved processes to streamline interstate licensing and credentialing requirements, while loosening online prescribing rules that currently inhibit telemedicine-based care. That progress at federal and state levels will then lead sleep telemedicine to more completely fulfill the promise it has held for more than 2 decades.

DISCLOSURE

The author has nothing to disclose.

REFERENCES

1. Waller M, Stotler C. Telemedicine: a primer. Curr Allergy Asthma Rep 2018;18(10):54.
2. Becker CD, Dandy K, Gaujean M, et al. Legal perspectives on telemedicine part 1: legal and regulatory issues. Perm J 2019;23:18–293.
3. Federation of State Medical Boards. Model policy for the appropriate use of telemedicine technologies in the practice of medicine 2014. Available at: https://www.fsmb.org/siteassets/advocacy/policies/fsmb_telemedicine_policy.pdf. Accessed January 30, 2019.
4. Watson NF, Rosen IM, Chervin RD, Board of Directors of the American Academy of Sleep Medicine. The past is prologue: the future of sleep medicine. J Clin Sleep Med 2017;13(1):127–35.
5. Venkateshiah SB, Hoque R, Collop N. Legal aspects of sleep medicine in the 21st century. Chest 2018; 154(3):691–8.
6. Brous E. Legal considerations in telehealth and telemedicine. Am J Nurs 2016;116(9):64–7.
7. Center for connected health policy. Available at: https://www.cchpca.org/telehealth-policy/credentialing-and-privileging. Accessed January 30, 2020.
8. Stupak B. H.R.6353 - Ryan Haight online pharmacy consumer protection Act of 2008. 2008. Available at: https://www.congress.gov/bill/110th-congress/house-bill/6353/text. Accessed January 30, 2020.
9. Singh J, Badr MS, Diebert W, et al. American Academy of Sleep Medicine (AASM) position paper for the use of telemedicine for the diagnosis and treatment of sleep disorders. J Clin Sleep Med 2015; 11(10):1187–98.
10. Chaet D, Clearfield R, Sabin JE, et al, Council on Ethical and Judicial Affairs American Medical Association. Ethical practice in telehealth and telemedicine. J Gen Intern Med 2017;32(10):1136–40.
11. Fleming DA, Edison KE, Pak H. Telehealth ethics. Telemed J E Health 2009;15(8):797–803.
12. Kobb R, Hoffman N, Lodge R, et al. Enhancing elder chronic care through technology and care coordination: report from a pilot. Telemed J E Health 2003; 9(2):189–95.
13. Marcin JP, Ellis J, Mawis R, et al. Using telemedicine to provide pediatric subspecialty care to children with special health care needs in an underserved rural community. Pediatrics 2004;113(1 Pt 1):1–6.
14. Aurora RN, Collop NA, Jacobowitz O, et al. Quality measures for the care of adult patients with obstructive sleep apnea. J Clin Sleep Med 2015;11(3): 357–83.
15. Kothare SV, Rosen CL, Lloyd RM, et al. Quality measures for the care of pediatric patients with obstructive sleep apnea. J Clin Sleep Med 2015;11(3): 385–404.
16. Krahn LE, Hershner S, Loeding LD, et al. Quality measures for the care of patients with narcolepsy. J Clin Sleep Med 2015;11(3):335.
17. Trotti LM, Goldstein CA, Harrod CG, et al. Quality measures for the care of adult patients with restless legs syndrome. J Clin Sleep Med 2015;11(3): 293–310.
18. Edinger JD, Buysse DJ, Deriy L, et al. Quality measures for the care of patients with insomnia. J Clin Sleep Med 2015;11(3):311–34.
19. Zulman DM, Chang ET, Wong A, et al. Effects of intensive primary care on high-need patient experiences: survey findings from a veterans affairs randomized quality improvement trial. J Gen Intern Med 2019;34(Suppl 1):75–81.

Telemedicine Coding and Reimbursement - Current and Future Trends

Fariha Abbasi-Feinberg, MD

KEYWORDS

- Telehealth codes • Telehealth reimbursement • Medicare telehealth • CPT telehealth codes
- Remote physiologic monitoring codes • Online digital evaluation codes • Telehealth legislation
- Non–face-to-face services

KEY POINTS

- Innovation in technology is redefining the world, including health care. Patients want convenient and quality interactions with their providers.
- The addition of telemedicine technologies and asynchronous provider-to-patient communications is creating a more connected model of health care that will improve access and the value of care while decreasing costs, as well as enabling patients to participate more directly in their own care.
- As new technologies and new models of care continue to emerge, providers need to continue to monitor the rapidly changing landscape of telemedicine coding and reimbursement.
- Telehealth coding and reimbursement rules are payor and state dependent.

Sleep disturbances affect an estimated 35% to 40% of the adult population in the United States. Approximately 5.9 million US adults have been diagnosed with obstructive sleep apnea, but 23.5 million Americans remain undiagnosed.[1] Among older adults, the prevalence of insomnia disorder, defined as difficulty initiating or maintaining sleep with daytime impairment, ranges from 25% to 40%.[2] Untreated insomnia and obstructive sleep apnea are associated with increased health care use and costs.[3]

Health care costs in the United States accounted for 17.8% of the gross domestic product in 2019. The US Centers for Medicare and Medicaid Services (CMS) projects that health care spending will reach 20% of gross domestic product by 2025.[4] Despite this financial outlay, the health outcome goals have not been achieved.

This failure may be attributable to a fragmented health care system as well as lack of access to care. The United States health care system has a serious workforce supply problem. The Association of American Medical Colleges (AAMC) projects that physician demand will continue to grow faster than supply, leading to a projected total physician shortfall by 2030 of between 40,800 and 104,900 physicians.[5] This shortfall includes sleep medicine specialists. Lack of access to care and cost of health care are leading to innovative models, including the growth of telehealth services. Sleep medicine is a technology-dense specialty and is poised to be active in telemedicine.[6,7]

Government and private payers appreciate the potential cost savings that are achievable through telemedicine. Medicare's focus on value-based

---

This article was accepted before the COVID-19 pandemic. Many of the coding guideline requirements have been temporarily suspended beginning March 6, 2020, and lasting through the national public health emergency as declared by the Secretary of Health and Human Services. Please see addendum for details. It is unclear at the time of this final submission how long these changes will stay in effect.

Millennium Physician Group, 13813 Metro Parkway, Fort Myers, FL 33912, USA

E-mail address: fabbasifeinberg@gmail.com

Sleep Med Clin 15 (2020) 417–429
https://doi.org/10.1016/j.jsmc.2020.06.002

care models has seen a significant shift from volume to value and led to an expansion of coverage for telemedicine-based services. The health care industry has realized that remote monitoring programs can be involved in chronic disease management and may be suitable for some acute medical scenarios as well. Many employer-based plans are contracting directly with physician groups to obtain health care that is convenient and efficient for the employees. The global telehealth market, which in 2016 was valued at $2.78 billion, is projected to reach $9.35 billion by 2021, growing at a compound annual growth rate of 27.5%.[8]

This excitement involving telemedicine is dampened by questions concerning reimbursement. Navigating issues regarding telehealth/telemedicine policy, coding, and reimbursement is complicated. CMS started reimbursing for telemedicine services in 1999 for some patients in rural areas but with significant limitations. Over the last few years there has been substantial expansion of coverage from CMS as well as commercial payors. This last year, 2019, has been active for telehealth legislation along with acceptance of new Current Procedural Terminology (CPT) codes.[9] There are slated changes coming in 2021 for Evaluation and Management (E/M) coding, along with new updates in remote patient monitoring and chronic care management guidelines. This article focuses on the CPT codes most pertinent to the practice of sleep medicine. Although every attempt is made to be accurate at the time of this writing, readers should understand that this is not a comprehensive list. Reviewing coding and reimbursement issues is an evolving situation and it is recommended that readers try to verify the most updated policies.

For the purpose of this analysis, telehealth coding and reimbursement has been divided into distinct categories (**Fig. 1**):

Medicare fee for service
Medicare advantage
Medicaid
Private payors
Employer pay
Self-pay

This articles review all these potential models of reimbursement with a focus on Medicare coding as the starting point. Whether these codes can be used by readers depends on the various payors, with Medicare having the strictest guidelines. Although readers may not meet all the Medicare rules for coding and reimbursement, many of the other entities described earlier allow these codes to be used for telehealth services.

DEFINITIONS

The terms telehealth and telemedicine are often used interchangeably. Telemedicine is usually defined as "the remote diagnosis and treatment of patients by means of telecommunication technology."[10] The Telehealth Resource Center defines telehealth as a "collection of means of methods for enhancing health care, public health and health education delivery and support using telecommunication technologies."[11] Telehealth is not a specific clinical service and is a more inclusive term for the wide collection of applications in the field. Telehealth may involve not only providers but also ancillary staff and health educators. Another term often heard is digital health, which includes categories such mobile health, health information technology wearable devices, telehealth, and telemedicine, as well as personalized medicine.

Table 1 provides some clarification of terms frequently used in this area of medicine. CMS defines telemedicine as live, interactive audiovisual transmission of a physician or other qualified health care provider (QHCP) from one site to another using telecommunication technology. There are detailed recommendations regarding the originating site, the distant site, and codes that can be billed. Asynchronous telemedicine, also known as store and forward, is only reimbursed by Medicare in certain states (Alaska and Hawaii) for specific situations.

MEDICARE

In almost all cases, Medicare only reimburses for live telemedicine interactions. The idea is to keep the contact similar to an in-person face-to-face visit. The Social Security Act governs which telemedicine services are and are not covered under Medicare. There are certain restrictions regarding eligible health care providers, and the locations of patients and services covered (**Table 2**).

The originating site must be located within a Health Professional Shortage Area or a county outside of a metropolitan statistical area. The Health Resources and Services Administration and the Census Bureau determine the eligibility[12] (https://data.hrsa.gov/tools/medicare/telehealth).

Patients need to be at 1 of 10 qualifying originating sites. Service is provided by 1 of 8 qualifying providers.

Technology is real time and face to face, and the service is among the list of CPT/Healthcare Common Procedure Coding System (HCPCS)[13] codes that are covered (CPT is Copyright 2019 American Medical Association. All rights reserved. CPT is a

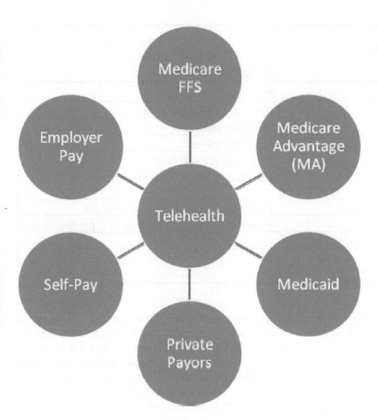

Table 1 Definitions	
Telemedicine (synchronous)	Telemedicine services are live, interactive audio and visual transmissions of a physician-patient encounter from one site to another using telecommunication technology
Distant site	The location of the physician or other qualified health care professional at the time the service is being furnished via telecommunication technology
Originating site	The location of a patient at the time the service is being furnished via a telecommunication system
Physician or Other Qualified Health Care Provider	Per CPT, a physician or other qualified health care professional is an individual who is qualified by education, training, licensure/regulation, and facility privileging who performs a professional service within their scope of practice and reports that professional service
Asynchronous telecommunication	Medical information is stored and forwarded to be reviewed by a physician or health care practitioner at a distant site. The medical information is reviewed without the patient being present. Also referred to as store-and-forward telehealth or noninteractive telecommunication

Table 2
Medicare telemedicine requirements

Location (Qualifying Rural)	Qualifying Providers
Physician or practitioner offices	Physicians
Hospitals	Nurse practitioners
Critical access hospitals	Physician assistants
Rural health clinics	Nurse midwives
Federally qualified health centers	Clinical nurse specialist
Hospital-based or critical access hospital—based renal dialysis center	Certified registered nurse anesthetists
Skilled nursing facilities	Clinical psychologist and sociologist
Community mental health centers	Registered dieticians or nutrition professionals
Mobile stroke units	—
Homes of patients with end-stage renal disease receiving home dialysis	—

registered trademark of the American Medical Association.) All the following codes can be found in the appropriate code books.

CURRENT PROCEDURAL TERMINOLOGY CODES FOR TELEMEDICINE

CMS recognizes and reimburses for certain CPT codes along with modifiers (**Table 3**). These codes include E/M codes as well as eligible CPT codes listed in the CPT manual.

Place of service (POS) is usually listed as 02 -Telehealth: the location where health services and health-related services are provided or received, through a telecommunication system.

(Note: This telehealth POS code does not apply to originating site facilities billing a facility fee.)

EVALUATION AND MANAGEMENT CODING FOR 2021

On November 1, 2019, CMS approved the Medicare physician fee schedule for 2020. This schedule includes a historic change in the way

physicians have been coding patient encounters for the last 25 years. These revisions to the E/M office visit CPT code changes will be effective January 1, 2021 and, because they will affect how physicians code for telemedicine E/M visits as well, the codes will be reviewed. Further changes may be described when the physician fee schedule is published for 2021, in the fall of 2020.

Summary of changes:[14,15]

1. Eliminate history and physical as elements for code selection. Providers need to perform a medically appropriate history and/or physical examination, which will contribute to the time spent with the patient as well as the medical decision making, but these "bullets" will not determine appropriate code level.
2. Documentation can be based on either medical decision making (MDM) or total time (TT)
   a. MDM uses the current CMS Table of Risk as groundwork for the new elements of MDM with some clarifications, including redefining some current concepts and data elements

Table 3
Modifiers

Modifier	Description
GT	Via interactive audio and video telecommunications systems
GQ	Via asynchronous telecommunications systems
95	Synchronous telemedicine service rendered via a real-time interactive audio and video telecommunications system (reported only with codes from Appendix P of CPT manual)
G0	Telehealth services for diagnosis, evaluation, or treatment of symptoms of an acute stroke

to focus on task for management of the patients (**Table 4**).

b. TT is the total minimum time the provider spends on date of service. This total includes non–face-to-face time, such as reviewing the chart, documentation, and care coordination (**Table 5**).

3. CPT code 99201 will be deleted, leaving 4 levels of new patient E/M codes but continuing with 5 levels of coding for established patients.

4. New add-on code for extended office visit time CPT code 99XXX and a new complexity add on code GPC1X.

Changes in terminology contrasted to familiar language (**Table 6**).

"Number of Diagnoses or Management Options" will become "Number and Complexity of Problems Addressed"

"Amount and/or Complexity of Data to be Reviewed" will become "Amount and/or Complexity of Data to be Reviewed and Analyzed"

"Risk of Complications and/or Morbidity or Mortality" will become "Risk of Complications and/or Morbidity or Mortality of Patient Management."

These E/M codes can be used for appropriate telemedicine visits with modifiers.

As an example, a patient is evaluated from the primary care physician's office in a rural setting as a follow-up visit for obstructive sleep apnea. The provider is at a distant site and performs appropriate follow-up visit for level 3 coding requirements. The provider would submit code 99213-GT. The originating site would also bill for a facility fee for hosting the patient (HCPCS code Q3014).

Medicare will reimburse the telemedicine service at the current fee schedule rate for the comparable in-person medical service.

MEDICARE-COVERED TECHNOLOGY-BASED SERVICES

Telemedicine policies are set by Congress with updates to the Social Security Act. A bill must be introduced and approved by both the House of Representatives and the Senate and signed into law by the President. This process occurs extremely slowly, if at all. Therefore, Medicare regulations for telemedicine are slow to change. Because of technological advancements, updates are essential. CMS has approved other options for various non–face-to face services that are covered and do not require any changes in legislation. These codes are included under the physician fee schedule and are updated on an annual basis. For 2020, the conversion factor is \$36.89. Work relative value units (RVUs) are not specifically covered in this review because they change on a yearly basis. CMS offers a free search tool for RVUs for every CPT code, as well as a jointly maintained site for HCPCS codes (https://www.cms.gov/apps/physician-fee-schedule/license-agreement.aspx, https://hcpcs.codes/search/).

NON–FACE-TO-FACE SERVICES
Online Digital Evaluation and Management Services

Online Digital Evaluation and Management Services are new additions to CPT inspired by new digital communication tools such as patient portals. These codes allow health care professionals to more efficiently connect with patients at home and exchange information. These new codes report online digital evaluation services or e-visits. These codes are patient initiated and are asynchronous. Consent is required from patients on an annual basis.

CPT 99421, 99422, and 99423 are patient-initiated services with physician or other qualified health care professionals (QHPs). These services require evaluation, assessment, and management

Table 4
Documentation for time or medical decision making

	Time		MDM	
Present	Typical face-to-face time	Number of diagnosis or management options	Amount and complexity of data to be reviewed	Risk of complications and/or morbidity or mortality
2021	TT on day of encounter	Number and complexity of problems addressed	Number and complexity of problems to be addressed	Risk of complications and/or morbidity/mortality of patient management

Table 5
Time for coding

E/M Code	Current Time (min)	Time in 2021 (min)
99202	20	15–29
99203	30	30–44
99204	45	45–59
99205	60	60–74
99211	5	NA
99212	10	10–19
99213	15	20–29
99214	25	30–39
99215	40	40–54

Abbreviation: NA, not applicable.

of the patients. They are not for communicating test results, scheduling appointments, and so forth. Each patient is an established patient and these services are initiated through a HIPPA (Health Insurance Portability and Accountability Act)-compliant platform. This service can occur over a period of 7 days and includes cumulative time to review records or data, develop a management plan, and communicate back to the patient. Online digital E/M services require a permanent document of the encounter and are performed by individuals who can bill for E/M services. They may not be used for work done by clinical staff.

CPT 99421: online digital E/M service for an established patient.
- Reported once for the cumulative time over a 7-day period
- Time includes review of the inquiry, review of records or data, and subsequent communication with the patient
- If a separately reported E/M visit occurs within the 7-day period, the time or complexity can be added to the reported E/M code
- From 5 to 10 minutes
CPT 99422: as above, 11 to 20 minutes
CPT 99243: as above, 21 or more minutes

The CPT editorial panel finalized similar codes for qualified nonphysician health care professionals (98970-98972), but these are not recognized by CMS. CMS has approved some G codes that can be used by qualified nonphysician health care providers, such as physical therapists, occupational therapists, social workers, dieticians, and speech therapists.

G2061: qualified nonphysician health care professional online assessment for an established patient
- Reported once for the cumulative time during the 7 days
- From 5 to 10 minutes
G2062: as above, for 11 to 20 minutes
G2063: as above, for 21 minutes or more

Table 6
Changes in terminology

Code	Level of MDM (2 out 3)	Number and Complexity of Problems Addressed	Amount and/or Complexity of Data to be Reviewed and Analyzed	Risk of Complications and/or Morbidity or Mortality of Patient Management
99211	NA	NA	NA	NA
99202 99212	Straightforward	Minimal	Minimal or none	Minimal risk of morbidity from additional diagnostic testing or treatment
99203 99213	Low	Low	Limited	Low risk of morbidity from additional diagnostic testing or treatment
99204 99214	Moderate	Moderate	Moderate	Moderate risk of morbidity from additional diagnostic testing and treatment
99205 99215	High	High	Extensive	High risk of morbidity from additional diagnostic testing and treatment

Virtual Care Codes

Physicians and QHPs can be reimbursed for these virtual check-ins for patients who are not certain whether their problems warrant an in-office visit. If the check-in does not lead to an appointment or is caused by a previous E/M visit within the last 7 days, these codes can be billed as a stand-alone service.

HCPCS G2012 virtual check ins

G2012: brief communication technology–based service (eg, virtual check-in) by a physician or other QHP who can report E/M services.

- Provided to an established patient
- Not originating from a related E/M service provided within the previous 7 days nor leading to an E/M service or procedure within the next 24 hours or soonest available appointment
- From 5 to 10 minutes of medical discussion
- No frequency or location requirements

HCPCS G2010 review of images or video

G2010: remote evaluation of recorded video and/or images submitted by an established patient (eg, store and forward).

- Including interpretation with follow-up with the patient within 24 business hours
- Not originating from a related E/M service provided within the previous 7 days nor leading to an E/M service or procedure within the next 24 hours or soonest available appointment

Once again, this can only be for established patients and involves interpretation of recorded images or videos and follow-up in 24 hours. Follow-up can be via phone call, audio/video, secure text, email, or patient portal communication.

DIGITALLY STORED DATA SERVICES/REMOTE PHYSIOLOGIC MONITORING AND TREATMENT MANAGEMENT SERVICES

These codes are used to report remote physiologic monitoring and treatment management services during a certain time frame. The devices used must be medical devices as defined by the US Food and Drug Administration (FDA) and the service must be ordered by a physician or QHP.

> CPT 99457: remote physiologic monitoring treatment management services are provided when clinical staff/physicians/other QHPs use the results of the remote physiologic monitoring to manage a patient under a specific treatment plan

- Twenty minutes of clinical staff (under general supervision), physician, or other QHP time in a calendar month
- Requires live, interactive communication with patient/caregiver during the month
- Can report once every 30 days

CPT 99458: remote physiologic monitoring treatment management services for additional 20 minutes

CPT 99453: initial setup and patient education on use of equipment

CPT 99454: FDA-approved device supply, recording and transmission of data

CPT 99091 was unbundled in 2018.

- This service is defined as collection and interpretation of physiologic data, stored and transmitted by the patient or caregiver to the physician or QHP
- This service requires an initial in-person visit and includes professional time involved with data acquisition, review, and interpretation and modification of care plan
- Including communication to patient or caregiver and appropriate documentation
- Time involved is 30 minutes every 30 days

CARE MANAGEMENT SERVICES

Sleep physicians may be involved with some of the care management services but probably not frequently. These new codes include Transitional Care Management, Chronic Care Management for 2 or more chronic conditions, as well as Principal Care Management Services for 1 chronic condition, which will most likely be used by specialists.

Principal Care Management Services

HCPCS G2064: chronic care management services for a single high-risk disease. Thirty minutes of physician or other qualifying health care professional time per calendar month with the following elements: 1 complex condition lasting at least 3 months, which is the focus of the care plan, the condition is of sufficient severity to place patient at risk of hospitalization, or has been the cause of a recent hospitalization; the condition requires development or revision of disease-specific care plan with frequent adjustments in the medication regimen and or the management of the condition is unusually complex because of comorbidities.

HCPCS G2065: As G2064, 30 minutes of clinical staff time, directed by a physician or other QHP.

INTERPROFESSIONAL TELEPHONE/INTERNET/ ELECTRONIC HEALTH RECORD CONSULTATIONS (CURRENT PROCEDURAL TERMINOLOGY 99446, 99447, 99448, 99449, 99451, 99452)

This is an assessment and management service requested by a treating physician or QHP for treatment advice from a physician with specific expertise to assist in the care of a patient without face-to-face contact between the patient and the specialist. This individual may be a new or an established patient with a new problem for the specialist. If this consult leads to a transfer of care, these codes are not reported. These codes include a verbal and written report. The different levels are based on the time of medical discussion and review: 5 to 10 minutes, 11 to 20 minutes, 21 to 30 minutes, or more than 31 minutes.

There is an updated list of covered Medicare telehealth services available at https://www.cms. gov/Medicare/Medicare-General-Information/ Telehealth/Telehealth-Codes.

Medicare Telehealth Changes for 2020 and Beyond

The Bipartisan Budget Act of 2018 was passed and has expanded stroke telehealth beyond rural areas. It also includes telehealth coverage to home and independent renal dialysis facilities.

The 2018 SUPPORT for Patients and Communities Act requires CMS to adjust their reimbursement policy for telehealth for treating individuals with substance use disorder or co-occurring mental health disorders by removing the geographic requirement for originating sites. This act went into effect January 1, 2020, with bundled-payment and intensity add-on codes.

The movement toward value-based care and reimbursement provides incentives for cost-efficient practices of care, including the resourceful use of integrated care teams. Alternative payment models, such as those included in Medicare Access and Chip Reauthorization Act of 2015, offer an opportunity to use telehealth services to meet the needs of providers and patients in this model of care. Certain bundled-payment programs and accountable care organizations are expanding how care is provided.[16] CMS continues to reconsider its limited definition of telehealth reimbursable services. The Creating Opportunities Now for Necessary and Effective Care Technologies (CONNECT) for Health Act of 2019 was introduced in the Senate in October 2019. This legislation acknowledges that use of telehealth services for Medicare patients is low. In particular, it notes that health care providers can furnish safe, effective, and high-quality care through telehealth and that barriers to the use of telehealth should be removed.[17]

The American Medical Association has formed a multistakeholder group called the Digital Payment Advisory Group, which is focused on coding and reimbursement issues for telehealth services.[18]

CMS accepts requests for new telehealth codes from any interested party, including medical specialty societies, individual providers, hospital systems, or state and federal agencies.[19] New telehealth codes are being added on a regular basis.

MEDICARE ADVANTAGE PROGRAMS AND ACCOUNTABLE CARE ORGANIZATIONS

Medicare Advantage plans allow private insurers an option to offer plans that are an alternative to traditional Medicare. Thirty-four percent of Medicare recipients are enrolled in a Medicare Advantage program, accounting for coverage of more than 23 million people.[20] In the past, Medicare Advantage programs could cover telehealth services only per the traditional Medicare guidelines. Section 50323 of the Bipartisan Budget Act of 2018 allowed for a significant change starting 2020 to allow Medicare Advantage programs to include delivery of telehealth services in a plan's basic benefit. It has eliminated the originating site rural restrictions and added patient homes as a qualifying originating site for certain Medicare Advantage plans, as well as accountable care organizations.[21]

This increased flexibility is allowing innovations to promote access to care in a more convenient and cost-effective manner. Many of the plans have developed state-of-the-art technology to ease the process for patients and providers. Most platforms include integration in electronic medical records. It is hoped that the promise of reimbursement for a wider range of telehealth services will encourage organizations to build up their infrastructure as older patients with physical limitations and lack of transport choose virtual visits as part of their health care.

Coding and reimbursement will be the same as in person, along with the modifiers.

MEDICAID

Medicaid is not tied to Medicare requirements. Each state has specific definitions and requirements. Telemedicine is viewed as a cost-effective alternative to the more traditional face-to-face way of providing medical care (eg, face-to-face consultations or examinations between provider and patient) that states can choose to cover. This definition is modeled on Medicare's definition of telehealth services (42 CFR 410.78). Note that the federal Medicaid statute does not recognize telemedicine as a distinct service.[22]

States are constantly updating and refining the policies. All 50 states have policies to allow and reimburse for certain Medicaid telehealth services.

The Center for Connected Health Policy (https://www.cchpca.org) has an up-to date Web site that monitors changes. At present, remote patient monitoring is available in about half of the states. Fewer states reimburse for asynchronous telemedicine (store and forward) but trends are in favor of these technologies.[23]

In contrast with Medicare policies, about 14 states allow the home as an eligible originating site and 16 states allow schools as an originating site (**Fig. 2**).

Medicaid reimbursement for specific states is unique. Particular questions to review include which services are covered, list of eligible providers, appropriate CPT codes, location restrictions for patient or provider, and whether a preexisting relationship is required between the patient and provider (https://www.americantelemed.org/; https://www.medicaid.gov/medicaid/benefits/telemedicine/index.html).

COMMERCIAL PAYORS

Telehealth laws for commercial payors can be divided in 2 categories. Coverage laws define whether a certain code is covered for a member. This contract is between the commercial payor and the consumer. Parity laws are between the health care plans and the providers.[24] These laws are independent contracts that define the reimbursement for services provided. Parity state laws require commercial payers to reimburse telehealth services the same way as in-person services (**Fig. 3**).

At the time of this writing, only 8 states do not have parity laws.[25] Ideally, both coverage and parity laws are required for an effective telehealth program.

The guidelines vary by state and payor and are constantly shifting as new policies are enacted. If

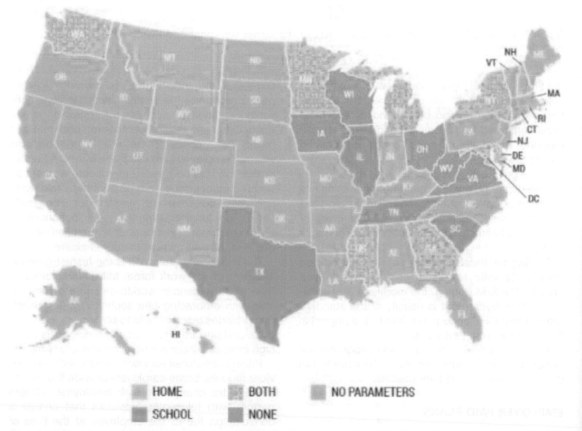

Fig. 2. Medicaid originating sites. (*Courtesy of* the Center for Connected Health Policy, Sacramento, CA; with permission.)

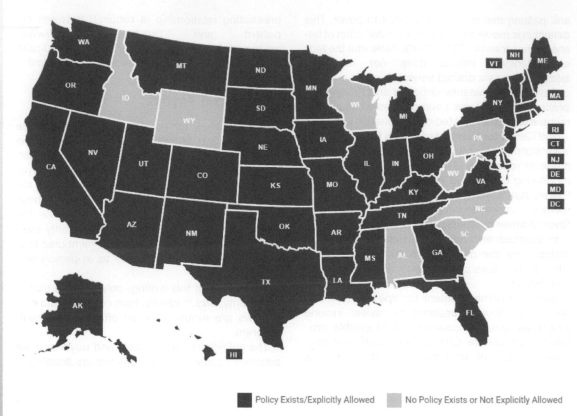

Policy Exists/Explicitly Allowed   No Policy Exists or Not Explicitly Allowed

Fig. 3. Parity laws for commercial plans. (*Courtesy of* the Center for Connected Health Policy, Sacramento, CA; with permission.)

the state has a telehealth parity law, any of the private payors should cover telehealth services. However, these are policy dependent and need to be confirmed for specific situations. It is recommended that insurance verification is obtained before the visits.

Some private payers still follow the more restrictive Medicare policy on location of originating site (location of patient) New updates are in progress to ease these restrictions to allow delivery of care to patients from any location (ie, home or work).

Coding for these visits is similar to Medicare coding. Specific telehealth codes can be used and, for the E/M coding, the modifier GT is applicable. Reimbursement is usually at the standard rate for that CPT code according to the physician fee schedule with that payer.

As the benefits of telemedicine programs are becoming more evident, many of the commercial payors are expanding their policies.

EMPLOYER-PAID PLANS

Many companies that sponsor group health care plans are offering telemedicine as part of their

coverage and this number is growing.[26] Companies recognize the benefits, which include convenience, better access for chronic health conditions, reduced absenteeism, and reduced health care costs. There are some concerns whether employees will use these benefits. Further instruction may be needed to educate workers on which medical issues are amenable to telehealth services and when to present for immediate care. Additional training may be beneficial to show employees how to access the telemedicine platform, as well as how to submit claims.

The millennial generation is the fastest-growing segment of the work force. Millennials comprise 50% of the American workforce and are comfortable with embracing new technology. Telehealth that provides quick access to physicians, personal data, and opportunity to research diagnosis has a high level of acceptability in this demographic.[27]

Pricing structures vary across telemedicine provider models. Some employers provide the benefit at no extra charge for their employees. Others partner with telehealth providers that charge a consultation fee to the employee at the time of visit. These fees create a barrier to employees using the service. Because telemedicine can potentially save employers money (especially those that are self-funded) from averted visits to doctors' offices, urgent care facilities, and emergency rooms, employers need a plan that encourages their employees to use their telehealth platform. There is some debate whether these services will reduce the cost of health care or just add to it.[28] This question will depend on the rate of use, and studies have shown clear cost savings of these programs.[29]

SELF-PAY

Thirty percent of telemedicine visits are paid out of pocket, according to a previous survey. This proportion compares with those who have visits covered by insurance (11%) or employers (10%).[30]

Telemedicine usage is most common among patients between 25 and 34 years of age; those more than 55 years of age are least likely to use telemedicine, according to a survey. However, more than half of those 55 years of age or older have accessed remote physician care through a phone call, which is considered a form of telehealth. Most of the patients surveyed, 76%, say that access to health care is more important than in-person appointments.[31]

There are numerous telehealth companies and platforms that are marketing direct to consumers because patients are willing to pay for the convenience. With telehealth, individuals can be evaluated for a sleep disorder, have a home sleep study, review results, and start treatment within a shorter time than it takes to see a sleep medicine specialist locally. This model is gaining popularity, especially among patients with a previous diagnosis of obstructive sleep apnea who need a new positive pressure device. Pricing is completely determined by the various parties involved.

SUMMARY

Innovation in technology is redefining the world, including health care. Patients want convenient and quality interactions with their providers. The addition of telemedicine technologies and asynchronous provider-to-patient communications is creating a more connected model of health care that will improve access and the value of care while decreasing costs, as well as enabling patients to participate more directly in their own care. As new technologies and new models of care continue to emerge, providers need to continue to monitor the rapidly changing landscape of telemedicine coding and reimbursement.

ADDENDUM

On March 13, 2020, the CMS announced sweeping changes allowing increased flexibility in delivering safe and effective care during the COVID-19 pandemic. These temporary modifications were made to encourage the use of telemedicine and eased previous requirements (discussed earlier). These constructive changes permit providers to continue to care for patients across the country in a safe and effective manner. Most private payors have also followed suit. The following is a review of the guidelines at the time of this final submission.

- One of the most important shifts includes coverage for telehealth services furnished in any health care facility but now also including the patients' homes.
- Many states have temporarily relaxed licensure requirements related to physicians licensed in another state and retired or clinically inactive physicians.
- Medicare has relaxed the restrictions related to providing telehealth and virtual services to new patients. For the duration of the public health emergency, telehealth and virtual services can be provided to new and established patients. Patients must consent, which may be obtained before or at the time of service. Ensure that consent is documented in the patient's medical record.
- Telemedicine visits are paid at the same rate as in-person visits. During the COVID-19 crisis, Medicare will pay the nonfacility amount for telehealth services when they are billed with the POS the physician would have used if the service had been provided in person (eg, POS 11: office). Physicians should append modifier -95 to the claim lines delivered via telehealth.
- CMS announced it will pay for telephone E/M visits (CPT codes 99441–99443) at parity with office E/M codes. On an interim basis, the RVUs and payment amounts will align as follows: 99441 will align with 99212, 99442 will align with 99213, and 99443 will align with 99214.
- During the COVID-19 emergency, Medicare will cover continuous positive airway pressure devices based on clinical assessment of the patient.

The COVID-19 pandemic has abruptly shifted the way clinicians practice sleep medicine. Telemedicine is suddenly not only convenient but necessary. It is unclear what the future of telemedicine coding and reimbursement will be once the pandemic resolves. Will clinicians return to all the previous stringent regulations? Will CMS and private payors appreciate the potential cost savings and benefits to patients and allow these temporary revisions to continue? Clinicians will have to await the answers.

DISCLOSURE

The author has nothing to disclose.

REFERENCES

1. Economic Impact of obstructive sleep apnea. American Academy of Sleep Medicine – Association for Sleep Clinicians and Researchers. 2019. Available at: https://aasm.org/advocacy/initiatives/economic-impact-obstructive-sleep-apnea/. Accessed December 2, 2019.
2. Wickwire EM, Vadlamani A, Tom SE, et al. Economic aspects of insomnia medication treatment among Medicare beneficiaries. Sleep 2019;43(1). https://doi.org/10.1093/sleep/zsz192.
3. Wickwire EM, Tom SE, Vadlamani A, et al. Older adult US Medicare beneficiaries with untreated obstructive sleep apnea are heavier users of health care than matched control patients. J Clin Sleep Med 2020;16(1):81–9.
4. CMS. US health care spending to reach nearly 20% of GDP by 2025. Advisory Board Daily Briefing. Available at: https://www.advisory.com/daily-briefing/2017/02/16/spending-growth. Accessed November 24, 2019.
5. New findings Confirm predictions on physician shortage. AAMC. 2019. Available at: https://www.aamc.org/news-insights/press-releases/new-findings-confirm-predictions-physician-shortage. Accessed January 2 , 2020.
6. Singh J, Badr MS, Diebert W, et al. American Academy of Sleep Medicine (AASM) position paper for the use of telemedicine for the diagnosis and treatment of sleep disorders. J Clin Sleep Med 2015;11(10):1187–98.
7. Watson NF. Health care savings: the economic value of diagnostic and therapeutic care for obstructive sleep apnea. J Clin Sleep Med 2016;12(08):1075–7.
8. Cohen JK. The growth of telehealth: 20 things to know. Becker's Hospital Review. Available at: https://www.beckershospitalreview.com/healthcare-information-technology/the-growth-of-telehealth-20-things-to-know.html. Accessed January 2, 2020.
9. CPT 2020 professional edition. Chicago: American Medical Association; 2019. CPT is a registered trademark of the American Medical Association.
10. mHealthIntelligence. Is there a difference between telemedicine and telehealth? mHealthIntelligence. 2019. Available at: https://www.mhealthintelligence.com/features/is-there-a-difference-between-telemedicine-and-telehealth. Accessed January 24, 2020.
11. National Consortium of Telehealth Research Centers. National Consortium of telehealth research Centers. Available at: https://www.telehealthresourcecenter.org/. Accessed December 2, 2019.
12. Telehealth Resource Centers (TRCs). Health Resources & services administration 2019. Available at: https://www.hrsa.gov/rural-health/telehealth/resource-centers. Accessed January 24, 2020.
13. CPT 2020. Professional edition. Chicago: American Medical Association; 2019.
14. Coders MBand. AMA Announces 2021 E/M changes. Medicalbillersandcoders. 2020. Available at: https://www.medicalbillersandcoders.com/blog/ama-announces-2021-em-changes/. Accessed January 20, 2020.
15. AMA issues checklist for the transition to E/M office visit changes. American Medical Association. 2019. Available at: https://www.ama-assn.org/press-center/press-releases/ama-issues-checklist-transition-em-office-visit-changes. Accessed January 30, 2020.
16. Tuckson RV, Edmunds M, Hodgkins ML. Telehealth. N Engl J Med 2017;377(16):1585–92.
17. Schatz Brian. Text - S.2741 - 116th Congress (2019-2020): creating Opportunities now for necessary and effective care technologies (CONNECT) for health Act of 2019. Congress.gov. 2019. Available at: https://www.congress.gov/bill/116th-congress/senate-bill/2741/text. Accessed January 29, 2020.
18. Digital Medicine Payment Advisory Group. American Medical Association. Available at: https://www.ama-assn.org/practice-management/digital/digital-medicine-payment-advisory-group. Accessed December 2, 2019.
19. Request for addition. CMS. Available at: https://www.cms.gov/Medicare/Medicare-General-Information/Telehealth/Addition. Accessed January 24, 2020.
20. Medicare advantage. The Henry J. Kaiser Family Foundation; 2019. Available at: https://www.kff.org/medicare/fact-sheet/medicare-advantage/. Accessed December 1,2019.
21. Press release CMS finalizes policies to bring innovative telehealth benefit to Medicare Advantage. CMS. Available at: https://www.cms.gov/newsroom/press-releases/cms-finalizes-policies-bring-innovative-telehealth-benefit-medicare-advantage. Accessed January 24, 2020.
22. Medicaid home. Medicaid home. 2020. Available at: https://www.medicaid.gov/. Accessed January 20, 2020.
23. Center for connected health policy. Thumbnail. Available at: http://www.cchpca.org/. Accessed January 24, 2020.
24. Resources. ATA. Available at: https://www.americantelemed.org/resource/. Accessed January 30, 2020.

25. Center for Connected Health Policy. Thumbnail. Available at: http://www.cchpca.org/. Accessed December 1, 2019.

26. The advantages of telehealth-powered employer Clinics. InTouch health. 2019. Available at: https://intouchhealth.com/the-advantages-of-telehealth-powered-employer-clinics/. Accessed January 2, 2020.

27. Millennials demand telehealth in a move away from traditional primary care model. Healthcare IT News. 2018. Available at: https://www.healthcareitnews.com/news/millennials-demand-telehealth-move-away-traditional-primary-care-model. Accessed January 30, 2020.

28. Licurse AM, Mehrotra A. The effect of telehealth on spending: thinking through the numbers. Annals of Internal medicine. 2018. Available at: https://annals.org/aim/article-abstract/2678087/effect-telehealth-spending-thinking-through-numbers. Accessed January 24, 2020.

29. Michaud TL, Zhou J, Mccarthy MA, et al. Costs of home-based telemedicine programs: a systematic review. Int J Technol Assess Health Care 2018; 34(4):410–8.

30. 2019 employer health benefits survey - summary of findings. The Henry J. Kaiser Family Foundation; 2019. Available at: https://www.kff.org/report-section/ehbs-2019-summary-of-findings/. Accessed January 26, 2020.

31. Vonk C. Telehealth trends to watch in 2020. GD - mobile telemedicine community paramedicine - general devices 2020. Available at: https://general-devices.com/telehealth-trends-to-watch-in-2020. Accessed January 16, 2020.

The Impact of Telehealth on the Organization of the Health System and Integrated Care

Cliona O'Donnell, MB BCh BAO[a,b], Silke Ryan, MD, PhD[a,b],
Walter T. McNicholas, MD, FERS[c,*]

KEYWORDS

• Telemedicine • Integrated care • Sleep medicine • Organization of the health system

KEY POINTS

- Prevalence of sleep-disordered breathing is growing and will need enhanced access to services and specialist input for a subset of patients.
- Telemedicine has potential to facilitate a move toward an integrated model of care, involving professionals from different disciplines and different organizations working together in a team-oriented way toward a shared goal of delivering all of a person's care requirements.
- A hub-and-spoke model of integrated care is likely to be the optimal organization of the health system with regard to sleep medicine.
- Telehealth has applications in all stages of the diagnosis, treatment, and follow-up of obstructive sleep apnea.
- Issues around consumer health technology and nonphysician sleep providers will need to be carefully evaluated in the development of a Telehealth system to promote integrated care.

INTRODUCTION

Sleep medicine is a rapidly developing field that is well-suited to initiatives such as Telehealth to provide safe, effective clinical care to an expanding group of patients. The optimal organization of the health system with regard to sleep medicine deserves special attention for a number of reasons: (1) the very high and growing prevalence of sleep disorders results in long waiting lists and a lack of specialist availability in many jurisdictions; (2) it has already integrated health technology to a greater degree than other fields, with potential to continue doing so; and (3) it involves a large burden of chronic disease that requires efficient diagnosis, commencement of treatment, and continuing follow-up. Thus, an integrated care approach involving multidisciplinary teams with input from both specialist and generalist sectors, centered around providing personalized care to the individual patient, is an appropriate and achievable goal in sleep medicine, especially with the use of health technologies and telehealth to aid integration.

Sleep-disordered breathing, of which obstructive sleep apnea (OSA) is the most prevalent disorder, accounts for a large proportion of the sleep medicine patient cohort. OSA remains underdiagnosed and undertreated, and patients with OSA

a UCD School of Medicine, Health Sciences Centre, University College Dublin, Belfield, Dublin 4, Ireland;
b Department of Respiratory and Sleep Medicine, St. Vincent's University Hospital, Elm Park, Dublin 4, Ireland;
c Department of Respiratory and Sleep Medicine, School of Medicine, University College Dublin, St. Vincent's University Hospital, St. Vincent's Hospital Group, Elm Park, Dublin 4, Ireland
* Corresponding author.
E-mail address: walter.mcnicholas@ucd.ie

Sleep Med Clin 15 (2020) 431–440
https://doi.org/10.1016/j.jsmc.2020.06.003
1556-407X/20/© 2020 Elsevier Inc. All rights reserved.

are at increased risk of hypertension, stroke, heart failure, diabetes, car accidents, and depression.[1] Sleep disorders affect an estimated 35% to 40% of the adult population in the United States, with a high cost burden, increased utilization of health care resources, and excess morbidity and mortality.[2] The HypnoLaus study published in 2015 involving 2168 subjects drawn from a Swiss general population and studied by home polysomnography (PSG) reported a very high prevalence for an apnea-hypopnea index (AHI) of 15 or more events per hour in 49.7% of men and 23.4% of women.[3] An AHI in the upper quartile of greater than 20.8 was independently associated with hypertension, diabetes, metabolic syndrome, and depression. The association of AHI with comorbidity is complicated by the finding that AHI rises with age,[4] whereas the association among OSA, hypertension, and cardiovascular disease is stronger in younger subjects, as is the relationship between OSA and relative mortality.[5] Furthermore, the AHI has also been shown to be poorly related to the classic symptoms of OSA, especially sleepiness.[6]

The preceding considerations illustrate the scale of the problem in the clinical assessment and management of patients with sleep-disordered breathing where personalized care is increasingly recognized as necessary to select the optimal treatment for the individual patient.[7] This review looks at the optimal organization of the health system to deliver the preceding goals, and how Telemedicine can facilitate the achievement of fully integrated care. It also will identify sleep-disordered breathing and other sleep disorders as specific examples of the potential for Telemedicine to improve integrated care.

OPTIMAL ORGANIZATION OF THE HEALTH SYSTEM TO PROMOTE INTEGRATED CARE IN SLEEP MEDICINE

The World Health Organization (WHO) defines integrated care as follows: Integrated Care is a concept bringing together inputs, delivery, management, and organization of services related to diagnosis, treatment, care, rehabilitation, and health promotion. Integration is a means to improve the services in relation to access, quality, user satisfaction, and efficiency. It involves professionals from different disciplines and different organizations working together in a team-oriented way toward a shared goal of delivering all of a person's care requirements.[8] Resources are shared, continuity of care is upheld, and the delivery process is integrated in the ideal system.[8]

Several driving forces are identified by WHO as pushing the development of integrated care among all health systems. These include demand-side factors, such as demographic change with an aging population, epidemiologic transitions, rising expectations, and patients' rights. Supply-side factors include the development of medical technologies and telemedicine, improving information systems, and economic pressures.[9]

Most of these factors are directly applicable to the field of sleep medicine. Sleep medicine is traditionally organized around specialist sleep centers that are referred patients whom they then diagnose and treat in-house, and communicate the outcomes back to the primary care referrer. Delivery of sleep services throughout Europe is limited by increasing prevalence associated with increasing age and increasing obesity, rising awareness of sleep disorders and the availability of consumer sleep technology, and improvement in available diagnostic services and information systems. The field of sleep medicine needs to evolve to meet these pressures, and movement toward a fully integrated system represents an optimal approach to the organization of health services in this context. Such integrated care involves collaboration among respiratory sleep specialists, neurologists, psychiatrists, otolaryngologists, dentists, and generalists at a medical level, and also integrating with physiologists, nurse practitioners, and industry providers to provide a cohesive, person-centered service. Such collaboration is likely to be greatly facilitated by tailored telehealth systems.

The move toward person-centered care should also be considered in the organization of the health system. This requirement includes improved communication, respectful and compassionate care of the individual, engaging patients in managing their own care, and integration of care.[10] Many health systems are currently fragmented, with poor communication of patient information between different health care providers. New ehealth technologies can support and link disjointed services across the continuum of care, such as improved electronic patient portals and the use of e-mail communication between patients and health care providers. The Health for All policy frameworks for the WHO European Region also addresses integration of services, with an emphasis on better access to family and community-oriented primary health care, supported by a flexible and responsive hospital system.[11]

As sleep also becomes more widely recognized as a pillar of health on a par with diet and exercise, more input will be required from generalists and improved referral pathways and communication with specialist services will be required. One qualitative study from 2012 found that sleep disorders are still underrecognized and not prioritized by generalists. They also found that communication between specialists and generalists in their jurisdiction was poor and led to a lack of interdisciplinary support for generalists in caring for patients with a sleep-disorder, as well as a lack of credibility for the sleep disorders specialty.[12] A recent study comparing the management of OSA by primary care physicians and specialist sleep physicians found no difference in the primary outcome of daytime sleepiness between groups after 6 months, nor in the secondary outcomes including quality of life measures, OSA symptoms, treatment adherence, and patient satisfaction. However, both diagnosis and treatment intervention in the 2 groups involved input from specialist nurses and training given to primary care physicians and nurses. They also had access to specialist support, which was availed of in a small number of cases. Furthermore, patients in this trial were deemed to be high risk for OSA based on screening, meaning that patients of uncertain diagnosis were not included in the study. This approach provides an example of a "hub-and-spoke"–type model in which access to specialist input is readily available, assisted by Telemedicine, and integrated with services provided by nurses with specialty training and industry. However, adequate resourcing and training are necessary to achieve the outcomes reported in this study.

The hub-and-spoke model ideally represents a network consisting of an anchor establishment offering a full array of services, complemented by secondary establishments that offer more limited service arrays (**Fig. 1**). Patients who need more intensive services can be re-routed to the hub for treatment.[13] The model is highly scalable and very efficient, and is well-suited to integration of care with the assistance of health technologies.

Another research initiative toward integrated care is SMART DOCS (Sustainable Methods, Algorithms, and Research Tools for Delivering Optimal Care Study).[14] This study uses a novel patient-centered outcomes and coordinated care management approach as a new outpatient care delivery model for patients with sleep disorders. The study uses novel technologies to integrate sleep medicine care among the well-informed patient, specialist, and referring clinician. The comprehensive procedures involved include a standardized screening/intake process involving a combination of previously validated screening tools in an online questionnaire, the use of home-based diagnostic technologies and treatment adherence monitoring, actigraphy and ambulatory blood pressure monitoring, and the co-management of patients with primary care together with enhanced patient-provider data, in addition to information sharing and education.[14]

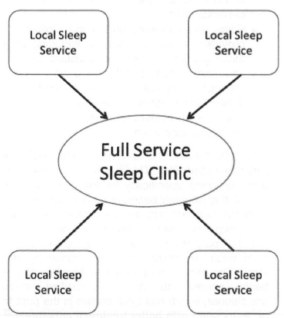

Local Sleep Service:
- Local hospital service with limited resources
- Primary Care
- Specialty services, eg, Dentistry, Otolaryngology

Full Service Sleep Clinic: Providing services for full polysomnography and related testing in addition to treatment and led by certified sleep specialist.

Fig. 1. Hub-and-spoke model of care.

These integrated procedures are greatly facilitated by telemedicine.

Thus, as seen in examples from Australia and the United States, the optimal organization of the health system with regard to sleep medicine will undoubtedly require the integration of Telemedicine to provide the most efficient, patient-centered, high-value care.

ROLE OF TELEHEALTH IN THE OPTIMAL ORGANIZATION OF HEALTH SYSTEMS

The European Commission has defined eHealth, or digital health, as follows: *The use of Information and Communication Technologies in health products, services and processes, combined with organizational change in health care systems and new skills, in order to improve health of citizens, efficiency and productivity in health care delivery, and the economic and social value of health.*[15] This definition clearly implies a key role for telehealth in the integrated organization of health care systems.

The American Telemedicine Association defines telemedicine as the use of medical information exchanged from one site to another via electronic communications to improve a patient's clinical health status.[16] and can be more broadly defined as the use of information and communications technology applications to provide health and long-term care services over a distance. In an ideal scenario, Telehealth should meet an urgent need for patient care provided at the prime point of need, favoring services in the home or in the community when possible. It offers the opportunity to deliver convenient, patient-centered, accessible care that overcomes many of the barriers present in traditional health care delivery systems, and should not simply be used as an adjunct to standard clinical care.[17] For the preceding reasons, telehealth care is a priority for Europe, as part of the "Digital Agenda for Europe," also for the UK National Health Service (NHS) as outlined in the "NHS Information Strategy," and for major health care providers in the United States such as the Department of Veterans Affairs.[18] However, most telehealth applications currently available remain segregated and require linking into more comprehensive eHealth strategies.[8]

The economic impact of telemedicine is complex to evaluate because there are different economic, social, and political factors at play. Most research studies have concluded that telemedicine systems are likely cost-effective but require better evidence.[18,19] A meta-analysis from 2008 reported that home monitoring was cost-effective in 21 of 23 studies,[20] but a report by Wootton[21] indicated a publication bias in telehealth studies looking at chronic disease management, with positive effects reported in 108 of 110 articles. Many telemedicine programs are still evolving from pilot-programs to full scale-up at regional and national levels. There is currently a lack of full assessment and evaluation of these programs, which will be essential in planning future telemedicine initiatives, as illustrated in one review of 17 telemedicine programs in Europe.[22] The development of these programs should be closely followed by those setting up sleep medicine telemedicine initiatives, as issues remain, such as confidentiality, data protection and ownership, financing, and quality of services.

The American Academy of Sleep Medicine (AASM) released a position paper on telemedicine in 2016,[2] recognizing the potential benefits and laying out conditions to promote optimal integration into clinical practice. Among other requirements, those applicable to the organization and integration of clinical care include the following:

- Telemedicine should adhere to standards of clinical care that mirror those of live office visits and include all aspects of diagnosis and treatment decisions as would be expected in a traditional encounter.
- Clinical judgment should be used to determine the scope and extent of telemedicine applications in the diagnosis of specific sleep disorders and patients.
- Live telemedicine visits should be recognized in a manner competitive or comparable with in-person visits.
- Roles, expectations, and responsibilities of providers should be defined, including both those at originating sites and distant sites.
- The care model should be a coordinated attempt to improve the value of health care delivery to the patient by sleep specialists, primary care providers, and other members of the health care team.

In 2016, the AASM also launched a telemedicine initiative called SleepTM,[23] a telemedicine platform designed specifically for the sleep field by AASM. It is primarily based around a secure video platform, but includes an interactive sleep diary and sleep log, sleep questionnaires, and the option for patients to import sleep data directly from wearable consumer sleep-monitoring devices. The aim of the program is to allow all patients access to a board-certified sleep practitioner, which has been shown in the past to be associated with better treatment adherence.[23]

Follow-up will also be facilitated with the SleepTM program, and given multiple studies have shown that consistent input is necessary to maintain continuous positive airway pressure (CPAP) adherence in OSA and thus treatment benefit, this is an extremely important facet of the program.

OBSTRUCTIVE SLEEP APNEA

Several studies have looked at the feasibility or cost-effectiveness of telemedicine in the management of OSA, with some contradictory results.[24] One Spanish study found that telemedicine did not result in improved CPAP compliance and resulted in lower patient satisfaction, but it was cheaper.[25] The Tele-OSA study found that tele-messaging alone and with tele-education improved CPAP compliance to what could be a clinically significant amount. The study in South Australia previously mentioned compared primary care and specialist input and found no difference in CPAP compliance between the 2 groups, but significant resources were available for both groups in terms of training provided to medical staff and patients.[26]

DIAGNOSIS

A health system that incorporates telemedicine to diagnose and treat a larger number of patients must be able to rely on accurate diagnostics as a fundamental part of management. In-laboratory PSG remains the gold standard for the diagnosis of sleep-disordered breathing, although home-based respiratory polygraphy is becoming more common and more widely available.[27] In-laboratory PSG is resource-intensive, limited by the availability of qualified staff, and expensive. A study in 2014 showed no significant difference between a 3-night home sleep study and PSG for patients without a high pretest probability of OSA.[28] It has previously been recommended that home sleep apnea testing not be used where there is ambiguity around the pretest probability or confounding comorbidities.[29,30] Masa and colleagues[29] reported that respiratory polygraphy is comparable to PSG for the diagnosis and therapeutic decision making for patients with a medium to high probability of OSA. However, data are frequently missing from home studies, which negatively affects their efficacy.[31]

Telemonitored PSG is a concept designed to overcome the disadvantages of home recordings, allowing dedicated technicians to verify the quality of the PSG recoding remotely in real time from a telemonitoring control panel. The protocols used to date have differed significantly and the evidence is therefore very weak.[31] However, a number of promising systems are attempting to overcome the problem of frequently missing data from conventional home studies.[27] As a screening tool, there are promising data looking at using nighttime pulse-oximetry telemedicine in patients at high risk for OSA.[31,32]

TREATMENT INITIATION

The treatment of OSA provides a challenge to ensure that patients can avail of specialist input when required. Mild OSA is often underrecognized in clinical practice and represents a management challenge as many different treatment options may be considered. The MERGE trial[33] involving 233 patients with mild OSA reported that quality of life significantly improved after 3 months in patients randomized to CPAP therapy compared with those randomized to supportive therapy. Notably, wireless monitoring was used to regularly review CPAP efficacy and adherence and may have helped to improve adherence.

These are patients who may not qualify for many of the studies evaluating home sleep apnea diagnosis but who may benefit from a trial of CPAP therapy. Conversely, their symptoms may not be attributable to their OSA, and inappropriate CPAP therapy may be avoided by referral to a specialist via telemedicine. A hub-and-spoke model may benefit this scenario whereby management decisions can be guided by sleep specialists and implemented by the local center. This was seen in the South Australian Primary Care study in which all patients in the Primary Care group commenced CPAP in contrast to only a proportion of patients in the Specialist group.[26] Also, mandibular advancement devices may be appropriate as an alternative to CPAP in certain subsets of patients with OSA.[34]

Phenotyping of OSA may improve the diagnosis of clinically significant OSA beyond the relatively imprecise measures of AHI and Epworth Sleepiness Scale and may benefit personalized diagnosis.[35] Gagnadoux and coworkers[36] identified 5 clusters, based on gender, presence of insomnia and comorbidities, depressive symptoms, and daytime sleepiness. CPAP use of more than 4 hours per night differed among the 5 clusters. This could provide additional prognostic information alerting the provider to those who may be at greater risk for nonadherence.[37]

Within the moderate-severe OSA group, there is established interest in the use of screening questionnaires, home sleep monitoring, and ambulatory management.[31] An initiative set up by the

Veterans Health Administration used video tele-conferencing, home sleep testing, modem-enabled positive airway pressure units, and auto-matically adjusting positive airway pressure ma-chines to set up a fully functional telemedicine-enabled sleep Medicine service that provides care to a large, geographically disperse group of veterans. In a prospective study, they compared this telemedicine service to standard in-person care and found no difference in automatic positive airway pressure adherence after 3 months and equal patient satisfaction between groups.[38]

FOLLOW-UP

CPAP is an effective treatment for OSA but bene-fits are heavily dependent on patient adherence,[37] and therapeutic benefits increase with higher num-ber of hours per night on therapy. However, compliance with CPAP is long-recognized as rela-tively poor in many studies and nightly compliance of more than 4 hours per night for 70% of days per week has been shown to vary between 30% and 60%.[8] Early adherence to CPAP usually predicts long-term adherence.[39] Compliance with CPAP is an area in which telemedicine is well-suited to optimization, with real-time wireless monitoring of CPAP use already available in many jurisdic-tions.[31] Patient's education, motivation, and active feedback can all have an impact on CPAP compli-ance. Conventional education and follow-up pro-grams are expensive and require active health staff involvement. Telemedicine should be useful in the area of CPAP adherence, although some studies have been equivocal on the benefit of certain programs.[27] CPAP adherence can be objectively and remotely measured in real time. Given that remote monitoring of health status is one of the objectives of telemedicine, wireless CPAP compliance monitoring is well-suited to an integrated care system.

A large recent randomized clinical trial looked at different approaches to using telemedicine to improve adherence. The study had 4 arms, looking at a tele-education program consisting of a Web-based OSA education, a CPAP telemonitoring pro-gram with automated feedback messaging, a combination of the 2, and usual care alone. Inter-estingly, this study found that the automated feed-back messaging improved CPAP compliance significantly, whereas the education program was not as beneficial. Sustained input from the tele-messaging service required limited provider input.[40] A similar outcome was found by a Cochrane review of educational, supportive, and behavioral interventions to improve CPAP adher-ence: Education alone improved adherence by only 35 minutes.[41] Furthermore, another study in Japan showed that long-term adherence rates to CPAP were improved with an intensive telemedi-cine follow-up program.[42] The HOPES study showed that in patients with sleep-disordered breathing after a stroke, a group in whom adher-ence is very challenging, a telemedicine interven-tion improved adherence rates in the short term at 3 months.[43] Overall, a consistent finding from studies of adherence is that sustained support and input from prescriber/clinician/nurse practi-tioner improves adherence and thereby improves outcomes.

Psychological measures of behavioral change constructs have been increasingly recognized as consistent predictors of CPAP adherence and as such, behavioral interventions have been most successful in optimizing adherence. However, these have not translated into routine care, primar-ily due to feasibility and cost issues.[44] Cognitive behavioral therapy (CBT) has been shown to be effective in small studies in improving adherence to more than 4 hours per night, and motivational enhancement therapy has also been shown to improve acceptance of but not adherence to CPAP up to a year. A Cochrane review found that behavioral therapy produces an improvement in nightly use of 1.5 hours, with a lack of cost-benefit data.[41] Given that CBT has been shown to be effective as a telemedicine-based interven-tion for insomnia and other sleep disorders,[45] and the resource-intensive nature of CBT for CPAP adherence, telemedicine is a potential op-tion to enhance delivery of such programs.

OTHER SLEEP DISORDERS

Sleep disorders other than sleep-disordered breathing are also frequently underdiagnosed, underresourced, and undertreated. Conditions such as insomnia and narcolepsy have a major impact on health, with effects on psychological and cognitive functioning and decreased quality of life. There is often a poor understanding of sleep disorders such as insomnia among primary care physicians and generalists.[46] Telehealth has been used for CBT with positive results in insomnia,[47,48] agoraphobia,[49] and posttraumatic stress disorder.[50] With regard to insomnia, Web-based programs have been shown to improve sleep quality, daytime fatigue, and overall severity of insomnia. A study of Web-based versus telehealth-based CBT found that both modalities provided clear benefit in the treatment of insomnia.[48] An integrated care hub-and-spoke model using telemedicine to access specialist advice and diagnostics from a hub, with subsequent easy referral to telemedicine-based CBT could streamline currently underresourced services for common but poorly understood sleep disorders, such as insomnia.

Patients with narcolepsy often remain undiagnosed for long periods after onset of symptoms and the condition is poorly understood by many general physicians. As understanding evolves of this disease, the need for access to specialist centers increases and telemedicine based on a hub-and-spoke model of care may facilitate such access. One study showed that patients ultimately diagnosed with narcolepsy were significantly more likely to have received a diagnosis in the category of mental disorders, nervous system disorders, and congenital anomalies before their diagnosis by a sleep specialist.[51] Narcolepsy was most often diagnosed by neurologists, with internists and general practitioners diagnosing narcolepsy much less frequently. .

CONSUMER HEALTH TECHNOLOGY

As interest in sleep as a pillar of health along with diet and exercise grows, consumer sleep technology utilization continues to increase. Sleep apps remain among the most popular apps downloaded for mobile devices. Patients sharing patient-generated health data with their sleep clinician is becoming more and more common. An understanding by the sleep specialist of the accuracy and utility of these technologies is expected from the patient. However, minimal validation data exist regarding the ability of consumer sleep technologies to perform the functions that they purport to. These devices are not subject to US Food and Drug Administration oversight and therefore cannot be relied on to make clinical decisions; however, it is likely that as these devices become increasingly sophisticated, some may undergo validation and ultimately have a role in clinical care, and therefore it is important to acknowledge them as adjuncts that may help with communication with patients, goal setting, and increasing active participation.[52]

Nonetheless, investment in consumer health technology dropped from a boom of US$1.3 billion in 2014 to $300 million In 2016, possibly reflecting a reality check in terms of what can be reliably achieved by consumer health technology without rigorous validation. A further concern Is the ownership of the data generated by consumer

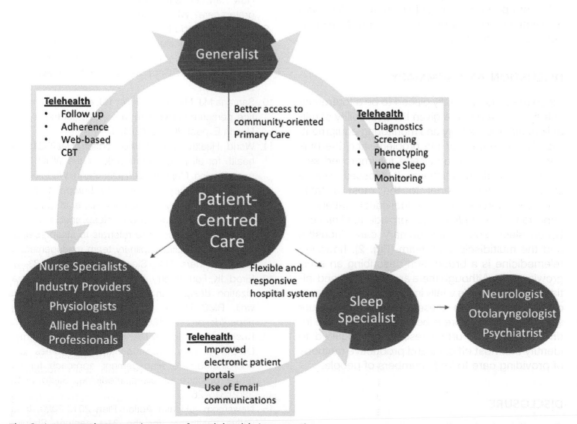

Fig. 2. Integrated care and targets for telehealth intervention.

wearables.[53] Currently these data are not owned by the generating patient, but often sold to third parties.

NONPHYSICIAN SLEEP PROVIDERS

In Australia, the sleep industry is unregulated and does not have a framework to govern or review emerging pathways in the community. Potential for conflict of interest has been noted within some pathways that offer both diagnostic and treatment services.[54] Community pharmacies have developed pathways that could provide access to sleep services to a large cohort of patients; however, given that they remain unregulated, there are difficulties with this approach. Many within the pharmacy community expressed concern over appropriate practices by some sleep providers, especially given that many services provide both diagnostics and access to long-term, potentially expensive treatment.[55] At a basic level, there must be concern that an industry provider that provides a diagnostic sleep service and also markets CPAP devices is more likely to recommend CPAP therapy even though alternative treatment modalities may be equally appropriate. Telehealth could be used to integrate these services offered with both primary care and sleep specialist care, allowing for a greater degree of objectivity in diagnosis and management.

DISCUSSION AND SUMMARY

Sleep medicine is ideally placed to be a forerunner in truly integrated care given the availability of reliable health technology and monitoring equipment, the chronic nature of the problem, and the burgeoning prevalence and need for improved services in most jurisdictions. It crosses several specialties, and referral to the most suitable specialist service for the individual patient is important. Telemedicine can provide the links between sleep specialists, primary care, industry, and the multidisciplinary team (**Fig. 2**); however, telemedicine is a broad term describing an ever-growing field. Although there are programs and initiatives in place, it is vitally important to continue to objectively evaluate these programs to ensure safe, high-quality care is being delivered to the individual patient. Further research is required to identify the most efficient and productive methods of providing care to large numbers of people.

DISCLOSURE

The authors have nothing to disclose.

REFERENCES

1. Hilbert J, Yaggi HK. Patient-centered care in obstructive sleep apnea: a vision for the future. Sleep Med Rev 2018;37:138–47.
2. Singh J, Badr MS, Diebert W, et al. American Academy of Sleep Medicine (AASM) position paper for the use of telemedicine for the diagnosis and treatment of sleep disorders. J Clin Sleep Med 2015; 11(10):1187–98.
3. Heinzer R, Vat S, Marques-Vidal P, et al. Prevalence of sleep-disordered breathing in the general population: the HypnoLaus study. Lancet Respir Med 2015; 3(4):310–8.
4. Senaratna CV, Perret J, Lodge C, et al. Prevalence of obstructive sleep apnea in the general population: a systematic review. Sleep Med Rev 2017;34:70–81.
5. Lavie P, Lavie L, Herer P. All-cause mortality in males with sleep apnoea syndrome: declining mortality rates with age. Eur Respir J 2005;25(3):514–20.
6. Deegan PC, McNicholas WT. Predictive value of clinical features for the obstructive sleep apnoea syndrome. Eur Respir J 1996;9(1):117–24.
7. Martinez-Garcia MA, Campos-Rodriguez F, Barbé F, et al. Precision medicine in obstructive sleep apnoea. Lancet Respir Med 2019;7(5):456–64.
8. Stroetmann KA, Kubitschke L, Robinson S, et al, How can telehealth help in the provision of integrated care? WHO Policy Brief, p. 39.
9. Gröne O, Garcia-Barbero M. WHO European Office for Integrated Health Care Services. Integrated care: a position paper of the WHO European Office for Integrated Health Care Services. Int J Integr Care 2001;1:e21.
10. Santana MJ, Manalili K, Jolley RJ, et al. How to practice person-centred care: a conceptual framework. Health Expect 2018;21(2):429–40.
11. World Health Organization, editor. Health21: the health for all policy framework for the WHO European Region. Copenhagen (Denmark): World Health Organization, Regional Office for Europe; 1999.
12. Hayes SM, Murray S, Castriotta RJ, et al. (Mis) perceptions and interactions of sleep specialists and generalists: obstacles to referrals to sleep specialists and the multidisciplinary team management of sleep disorders. J Clin Sleep Med 2012;8(6):633–42.
13. Elrod JK, Fortenberry JL. The hub-and-spoke organization design: an avenue for serving patients well. BMC Health Serv Res 2017;17(Suppl 1). https://doi.org/10.1186/s12913-017-2341-x.
14. Kushida CA, Nichols DA, Holmes TH, et al. Smart DOCS: a new patient-centered outcomes and coordinated-care management approach for the future practice of sleep medicine. Sleep 2015; 38(2):315–26.
15. Newsroom, eHealth Action Plan 2012-2020: Innovative healthcare for the 21st century, Shaping

Europe's digital future - European Commission. Available at: https://ec.europa.eu/digital-single-market/en/news/ehealth-action-plan-2012-2020-innovative-healthcare-21st-century. Accessed February 24, 2020.

16. Voran D. Telemedicine and beyond. Mo Med 2015; 112(2):129–35.

17. Dinesen B, Nonnecke B, Lindeman D, et al. Personalized telehealth in the future: a global research agenda. J Med Internet Res 2016;18(3). https://doi.org/10.2196/jmir.5257.

18. McLean S, Sheikh A, Cresswell K, et al. The impact of telehealthcare on the quality and safety of care: a systematic overview. PLoS One 2013;8(8).

19. de la Torre-Díez I, López-Coronado M, Vaca C, et al. Cost-utility and cost-effectiveness studies of telemedicine, electronic, and mobile health systems in the literature: a systematic review. Telemed J E Health 2015;21(2):81–5.

20. Sv R, Mp G. A systematic review of the key indicators for assessing telehomecare cost-effectiveness. Telemed J E Health 2008;14(9):896–904.

21. Wootton R. Twenty years of telemedicine in chronic disease management – an evidence synthesis. J Telemed Telecare 2012;18(4):211–20.

22. Baltaxe E, Czypionka T, Kraus M, et al. Digital health transformation of integrated care in Europe: overarching analysis of 17 integrated care programs. J Med Internet Res 2019;21(9):e14956.

23. Watson NF. Expanding patient access to quality sleep health care through telemedicine. J Clin Sleep Med 2016;12(2):155–6.

24. Lugo VM, Garmendia O, Suarez-Giron M, et al. Comprehensive management of obstructive sleep apnea by telemedicine: clinical improvement and cost-effectiveness of a Virtual Sleep Unit. A randomized controlled trial. PLoS One 2019;14(10). https://doi.org/10.1371/journal.pone.0224069.

25. Turino C, Batlle J, Woehrle H, et al. Management of continuous positive airway pressure treatment compliance using telemonitoring in obstructive sleep apnoea. Eur Respir J 2017;49(2). https://doi.org/10.1183/13993003.01128-2016.

26. Chai-Coetzer CL, Antic NA, Rowland LS, et al. Primary care vs specialist sleep center management of obstructive sleep apnea and daytime sleepiness and quality of life: a randomized trial. JAMA 2013; 309(10):997–1004.

27. Bruyneel M. Telemedicine in the diagnosis and treatment of sleep apnoea. Eur Respir Rev 2019;28(151). https://doi.org/10.1183/16000617.0093-2018.

28. Guerrero A, Embid C, Isetta V, et al. Management of sleep apnea without high pretest probability or with comorbidities by three nights of portable sleep monitoring. Sleep 2014;37(8):1363–73.

29. Masa JF, Corral J, Pereira R, et al. Therapeutic decision-making for sleep apnea and hypopnea syndrome using home respiratory polygraphy: a large multicentric study. Am J Respir Crit Care Med 2011;184(8):964–71.

30. Masa JF, Corral J, Sanchez de Cos J. Effectiveness of three sleep apnea management alternatives. Available at: https://www.ncbi.nlm.nih.gov/pmc/articles/PMC3825429/. Accessed: February 19, 2020.

31. Verbraecken J. Telemedicine applications in sleep disordered breathing: thinking out of the box. Sleep Med Clin 2016;11(4):445–59.

32. Chai-Coetzer CL, Antic N, Rowland L, et al. A simplified model of screening questionnaire and home monitoring for obstructive sleep apnoea in primary care. Thorax 2011;66(3):213–9.

33. Wimms AJ, Kelly JL, Turnbull CD, et al. Continuous positive airway pressure versus standard care for the treatment of people with mild obstructive sleep apnoea (MERGE): a multicentre, randomised controlled trial - the Lancet Respiratory Medicine. Available at: https://www.thelancet.com/journals/lanres/article/PIIS2213-2600(19)30402-3/fulltext. Accessed January 31, 2020.

34. Bratton DJ, Gaisl T, Schlatzer C, et al. Comparison of the effects of continuous positive airway pressure and mandibular advancement devices on sleepiness in patients with obstructive sleep apnoea: a network meta-analysis. Lancet Respir Med 2015; 3(11):869–78.

35. Sânchez-de-la-Torre M, Gozal D. Obstructive sleep apnea: in search of precision. Expert Rev Precis Med Drug Dev 2017;2(4):217–28.

36. Gagnadoux F, et al. Relationship Between OSA Clinical Phenotypes and CPAP Treatment Outcomes. Chest 149; 1:288–90.

37. Weaver TE. Novel aspects of CPAP treatment and interventions to improve CPAP adherence. J Clin Med 2019;8(12). https://doi.org/10.3390/jcm8122220.

38. Fields BG, Behari P, McCloskey S, et al. Remote ambulatory management of veterans with obstructive sleep apnea. Sleep 2016;39(3):501–9.

39. Weaver TE, Kribbs NB, Pack A, et al. Night-to-night variability in CPAP use over the first three months of treatment. Sleep 1997;20(4):278–83.

40. Hwang D, Chang JW, Benjafield AV, et al. Effect of telemedicine education and telemonitoring on continuous positive airway pressure adherence. the Tele-OSA randomized trial. Am J Respir Crit Care Med 2017;197(1):117–26.

41. Wozniak DR, Lasserson TJ, Smith I. Educational, supportive and behavioural interventions to improve usage of continuous positive airway pressure machines in adults with obstructive sleep apnoea. Cochrane Database Syst Rev 2014;(1):CD007736.

42. Murase K, Tanizawa K, Minami T, et al. A randomized controlled trial of telemedicine for long-term sleep apnea CPAP management. Ann

Am Thorac Soc 2019. https://doi.org/10.1513/AnnalsATS.201907-494OC.

43. Kotzian ST, Saletu M, Schwarzinger A, et al. Proactive telemedicine monitoring of sleep apnea treatment improves adherence in people with stroke– a randomized controlled trial (HOPES study). Sleep Med 2019;64:48–55.

44. Bakker JP, Weaver TE, Parthasarathy S, et al. Adherence to CPAP: what should we be aiming for, and how can we get there? Chest 2019; 155(6):1272–87.

45. Seyffert M, Lagisetty P, Landgraf J, et al. Internet-delivered cognitive behavioral therapy to treat insomnia: a systematic review and meta-analysis. PLoS One 2016;11(2). https://doi.org/10.1371/journal.pone.0149139.

46. Khawaja IS, Hurwitz TD, Herr A, et al. Can primary care sleep medicine integration work? Prim Care Companion CNS Disord 2014;16(no. 2). https://doi.org/10.4088/PCC.13br01593.

47. Espie CA, Kyle SD, Williams C, et al. A randomized, placebo-controlled trial of online cognitive behavioral therapy for chronic insomnia disorder delivered via an automated media-rich web application. Sleep 2012;35(6):769–81.

48. Holmqvist M, Vincent N, Walsh K. Web- vs telehealth-based delivery of cognitive behavioral therapy for insomnia: a randomized controlled trial. Sleep Med 2014;15(2):187–95.

49. Bouchard S, Paquin B, Payeur R, et al. Delivering cognitive-behavior therapy for panic disorder with agoraphobia in videoconference. Telemed J E Health 2004;10(1):13–25.

50. Frueh BC, Monnier J, Yim E, et al. A randomized trial of telepsychiatry for post-traumatic stress disorder. J Telemed Telecare 2016. https://doi.org/10.1258/135763307780677604.

51. Kryger MH, Walid R, Manfreda J. Diagnoses received by narcolepsy patients in the year prior to diagnosis by a sleep specialist. Sleep 2002;25(1):36–41.

52. Khosla S, Deak MC, Gault D, et al. Consumer sleep technology: an American Academy of Sleep Medicine Position Statement. J Clin Sleep Med 2018;14(05):877–80.

53. Piwek L, Ellis DA, Andrews S, et al. The rise of consumer health wearables: Promises and barriers. PLoS Med 2016;13(2). https://doi.org/10.1371/journal.pmed.1001953.

54. Hanes CA, Wong KKH, Saini B. Diagnostic pathways for obstructive sleep apnoea in the Australian community: observations from pharmacy-based CPAP providers. Sleep Breath 2015;19(4):1241–8.

55. Hanes CA, Wong KKH, Saini B. Consolidating innovative practice models: the case for obstructive sleep apnea services in Australian pharmacies. Res Soc Adm Pharm 2015;11(3):412–27.

Impact of Telehealth on Health Economics

Burton N. Melius, MBA[a],*, Walter D. Conwell, MD, MBA[b]

KEYWORDS

- Telehealth • Patient engagement • Health economics • Care delivery

KEY POINTS

- As part of an efficient, continuously improving care delivery system, telehealth can increase patient engagement by creating new or additional ways of communicating with patients' physicians.
- Telehealth has the potential to increase patient and primary care provider access to specialists, provide specialist support to rural providers, assist with on-going monitoring and support for patients with chronic conditions, and reduce health care expenses by maximizing the use of specialists without the need to duplicate coverage in multiple locations.
- Current and future physicians will need to develop competencies that will enable them to navigate this new telehealth landscape.

With the recent outbreak of the COVID-19 pandemic, health care organizations were forced to change the way they delivery care quickly. The pandemic caused many previously existing barriers to fall quickly in the need to be able to provide care safely and effectively, while at the same time preserving scare resources for patients in need. The expansion of telehealth services was a solution that could be implemented and/or expanded quickly and that met both of those criteria.

There has been a desire by health care organizations to shift the delivery of health care from higher cost settings to lower cost settings (eg, from the main operating room to ambulatory surgery centers) and to bring care from the hospital to community settings so it is closer to home for patients. Telemedicine is a vehicle that allows care delivery to stay closer to home, whether it is in a rural clinic far from a major metropolitan area or a smaller community hospital that may not have a specialist on site. Telemedicine allows rural clinics or community hospitals to connect with specialists anywhere in the world and receive consultative support and even care oversight by the specialist or a team of specialists.[1,2]

Moving toward an effective, efficient, and continuously improving health system is an important goal for the US health care system, allowing it to contain costs while providing safe care with high-quality outcomes.[1] In 2018, health care spending in the United States reached $3.6 trillion or $11,172 per person. This figure equates to 17.7% of the gross domestic product[3] (for comparison, in 2017, the United Kingdom spent $3,858, Japan spent $4,169, Canada spent $4755, and France spent $4380; the United States was at $10,246 in 2017 based on data from The World Bank from 2019). Even with this high rate of health care spending per capita, according to a recent data release by the Centers for Disease Control and Prevention, the United States ranked 55th in the world for maternal mortality, which is a sentinel public health indicator.[4]

As part of an efficient, continuously improving care delivery system, telehealth can increase patient engagement by creating new or additional ways of communicating with patients' physicians.

[a] Southern California Permanente Medical Group, East Walnut Street, Pasadena, CA 91188, USA;
[b] Department of Clinical Science, Kaiser Permanente Bernard J. Tyson School of Medicine, 98 South Los Robles Avenue, Pasadena, CA 91101, USA
* Corresponding author.
E-mail address: Burton.N.Melius@kp.org

Sleep Med Clin 15 (2020) 441–447
https://doi.org/10.1016/j.jsmc.2020.06.005
1556-407X/20/© 2020 Elsevier Inc. All rights reserved.

In the landmark report by the Institute of Medicine (IOM) titled *Crossing the Quality Chasm: A New health System for the 21st Century*, patient-centeredness was listed as 1 of the 6 aims for health care improvement. Patient-centeredness was defined as "respectful of and responsive to individual patient preferences, needs, and values and ensuring that patient values guide all clinical decisions."[5] In 2012 the IOM followed up with *Best Care at Lower Cost: The Path to Continuously Learning Health Care in America*. In this report, they listed 7 characteristics of an effective, efficient, and continuously improving health system of which one is "engaged, empowered patients."[5] Increased patient engagement is associated with better health outcomes, a better care experience, and lower health care costs.

Families indicate that patients want their providers to take a holistic, rather than a disease-based, approach to their care. They want clinicians to coordinate their care and communicate effectively across care settings. They want tools to help them manage their health conditions. Patients see efforts to engage them in their care as a path toward shared decision making and getting help from their clinicians in better understanding their health conditions. Of the patients surveyed who reported having 1 or more chronic conditions, almost all agreed that their care should be well coordinated, but only half reported that their care actually was coordinated. The question for many health care executives now is how to build a patient-centered health care system and deliver high-quality care in ways that are beneficial for both their patients and their bottom lines.[5]

This article explores areas where telehealth can provide value in the care delivery system, how to assess the value of telemedicine, ways of completing an economic analysis, and the role of telemedicine in medical education.

WHAT VALUE CAN TELEHEALTH PROVIDE

Telehealth has the potential to increase patient and primary care provider access to specialists, provide specialist support to rural providers, assist with on-going monitoring and support for patients with chronic conditions, and reduce health care expenses by maximizing the use of specialists without the need to duplicate coverage in multiple locations. Telemedicine has already been implemented for patients who live remotely, have limited access to specialists, or may have chronic conditions that require regular monitoring. Examples include monitoring care for patients with heart conditions or diabetes through the transmissions of echocardiograms for faster expert diagnosis and the frequent monitoring of patients with diabetes or heart failure via telephone or videoconference. In dermatology and ophthalmology, videoconferencing and image transmission allow long-distance consultations with experts for faster diagnosis and treatment while also avoiding travel costs for patients and families.[2]

Telehealth opens the door to many streams of communication among patients and clinicians and creates opportunities for patients to become engaged in their health care planning. New telehealth capabilities also improve patient engagement. Structured help lines, telemonitoring of physiologic data such as weight and blood pressure, and telecoaching in order to provide patients with structured after-care contact with clinicians can improve patients' decision making, confidence, and satisfaction. Recognizing the transformative potential of patient-engaged care, new methods of organizing and paying for health care tie reimbursement to performance based on measures of patient satisfaction and engagement.[5]

ASSESSING THE ECONOMIC IMPACT OF TELEHEALTH

To understand the true value of telehealth for an organization, it is necessary to understand the value telehealth will bring. This understanding requires some type of economic evaluation where the costs and consequences of telemedicine can be identified, measured, and compared with any alternatives. In the case of telemedicine, the alternatives normally include the conventional system of delivering health care and telemedicine. A comparison would allow a decision to be made on which option represents the best use of organizational resources.[6] This decision is essential because there are typically limited resources that are unable to meet all the needs without driving an organization into debt, so choices must be made as to how limited resources will be allocated.[6] Understanding and applying economic methods in health research is vital to promote the efficiency and sustainability of health care, one of the core goals that telehealth aims to achieve.[7]

As mentioned earlier, economic evaluations provide information about whether health care technologies represent an efficient use of resources by comparing the costs and benefits of one health care technology with another. Because health care budgets are limited, resources should be allocated to technologies where the ratio of incremental costs to incremental benefits lies within a given cost-effectiveness threshold. This ratio (or threshold) represents the society's willingness to pay for an additional unit of health.[8] Given the innovative nature of telehealth interventions and the dynamic nature of technology, conducting an economic analysis in this area should involve the incorporation of societal values and the preferences of users, something that is possible with cost-benefit analysis.[7]

As part of the assessment of the economic value of telemedicine, it is necessary to estimate the economic benefits to a program. To do this, it is helpful to look at it from the client or patient's perspective, the physician or health care provider's perspective, and the perspective of any other stakeholders. From the patient's perspective, there is (1) increased access to health care, (2) faster and potentially more accurate diagnosis and treatment, (3) reduced waiting time, (4) increased medication adherence, (5) an increased ability for self-care, (6) avoided travel expenditures, and (7) decreased risk of job loss or time away from work. The first 4 of these benefits have the additional potential benefit of reduced morbidity and possible avoided mortality.[2,7]

Looking at the benefits from the physician or provider's perspective, there might be (1) avoided office visits, (2) increased medication adherence, (3) easier and increased knowledge transfer among practitioners, (4) increased accuracy and faster diagnosis, (5) increased patient satisfaction, and (6) clinical confirmation (second opinion). These benefits may be a mixed bag for physicians; the patients can access them faster through telehealth but the physicians may lose revenue because of avoided office visits.[2,6]

Other stakeholders may include the hospital, the insurer, pharmaceutical companies, and the employer. As an example, the hospital may see reduced length of stay, avoided readmissions, avoided emergency room visits, and even avoided hospitalizations. These things need to be accounted for in the economic analysis. From the hospital perspective, these may not necessarily be positive things because they may drive down revenue, although they may be offset by increased quality outcomes driven by telehealth consults with distant specialists that ultimately have a positive impact on the reputation and brand of the hospital. Although the reduced hospital stays or admissions may decrease revenue in the short term, the increased recognition of high-quality outcomes could increase revenue in the long term through additional contracts with other insurers. The benefits to other stakeholders are fewer, but, for employers, it may mean less time off needed for workers so there is less of a loss of productivity. There is the possibility of increased or easier access to health care for a special population; for example, prisoners.[2] It is important to consider all stakeholders and ensure an adequate understanding of the benefits of telemedicine from their perspectives.

There are 2 additional points to consider when conducting an economic evaluation. In terms of telemedicine, the technology is changing rapidly. In a 2013 article in the *MIT News* on predicting the progress of technology, research showed that Moore's Law and Wright's Law best predict how technology improves. Moore's Law states that the number of components on a computer chip double every 18 months. Wright's Law states that the rate of improvement increases exponentially over time.[9] The implication of these 2 laws is evident in telemedicine because any lessons and conclusions derived from economic evaluations of telemedicine programs may lose validity in a short period of time because of the rapid and continuous decline in equipment prices caused by continuously improving and changing technology.[2]

The second point to consider when conducting a cost analysis is whether the costs and consequences of interventions and their alternatives can be adapted from one context to another.[1] Although this is not the primary consideration, there is value in considering this, particularly in a larger organization where there may be multiple projects in subsequent years. Being able to generalize results against other analyses allows comparison with other organizations and across settings internally to an organization.[1] Rigorous benefit-cost analyses of telemedicine programs could provide credible and comparative evidence of their economic viability and thus lead to the adoption and/or expansion of the most successful programs. As part of the analysis, it would be important to show that telehealth strategies can help slow the growth of health care spending without compromising access, effectiveness, and safety.[2] Tailoring analysis methods appropriately to the intervention and context is vital to produce findings that can be generalized outside of the research environment.[7]

TYPES OF ECONOMIC EVALUATION

The type of analysis to be used often depends on the business question to be answered. In the case of telemedicine, the question may be whether it is less expensive to insert telemedicine into an existing care pathway, replace an existing process, or introduce a completely new service. If investing in telemedicine costs more and is more effective, the decision maker would need information on how much more beneficial it is for the costs involved.[1] If specific outcome measures show equal or better patient outcomes than usual care, then the next step is to assess the differences in costs using standard costing techniques. However, lower cost is not always the best path of action. In addition, clinical outcomes may be better with a combination of traditional approach and telemedicine, even if that leads to a higher cost. There may be additional components of the economic evaluation that are challenging to place a value on but are important considerations. For example, better quality outcomes may lead to increased market share, potential good will with the community, and peer recognition as a leader in high-quality health care delivery. On the reverse side, this type of recognition may lead to what is known as adverse selection, where sicker patients, or patients with more challenging chronic conditions and complex situations, may choose to use services. These positive and challenging situations need to be accounted for in any economic analysis.

To complicate things further, there are several categories of costs that need to be accounted for. Fixed costs account for things like equipment/technology, office space, and depreciation. Variable costs cover maintenance and repairs, telecommunication costs, administrative support, supplies, training, and wages for staff and technicians. There may even be additional costs such as marketing or travel.[2] From a cost perspective, telehealth interventions have been shown to reduce mortality and hospitalizations for patients with chronic heart disease.[5] Each type of analysis has strengths and weaknesses when it comes to accounting for costs and intangibles such as good will and adverse selection.

Three of the most common economic evaluation methods are cost analysis, cost-effectiveness analysis, and benefit-cost analysis. What follows is a short description of each.[2,6,7]

Cost Analysis

This type of evaluation is the most basic, assessing the costs associated with the service, any potential cost savings, plus any changes in revenue. This type of analysis is typically a comparison of multiple options that cost out different variations of how to deliver the service. The assumption is that the options will all have similar results. This type of evaluation typically does not include an analysis of the options. It may include some aspect of the cost of the outcome; for example, one option may have a longer length of stay in an inpatient setting than another. However, it typically does not include an analysis of the quality of one outcome compared with another.

Cost-Effectiveness Analysis

Cost-effectiveness analysis (CEA) is a more inclusive evaluation in that it considers both costs and outcomes. This type of analysis evaluates both the costs and outcomes of the program and expresses the results as a cost per unit of outcome. Although a CEA evaluation is more comprehensive in that it includes outcomes, it does have a drawback in that it is only able to evaluate a single outcome.

Benefit-Cost Analysis

This is the most comprehensive of the 3 types of cost analysis. The benefit-cost analysis allows the evaluation of options with multiple outcomes. It takes the benefits of the option and quantifies them by placing a monetary value that then can be combined with the costs. This approach allows a more equal comparison with other options to determine whether a program is economically justified and better than alternative uses of the same resources. In addition, the costs and benefits are discounted to account for the present value of the future costs and benefits, which allows for comparison across options that have different periods of time. It allows for the comparison of one option that may start this year with other options that start in different years. The dollars in future years will have been inflated by a specific percentage to account for average inflation, but then discounted back to current value to allow an "apples-with-apples" comparison of options.

Cost-Utility Analysis

The cost-utility analysis is the most comprehensive of the economic evaluation models and is considered the gold standard because it captures the value of the gains in health-related quality of life. Although it is the most comprehensive, it may also be challenging to use because telehealth interventions are frequently intended to provide greater efficiency, convenience, and access for patients and it may be difficult or unrealistic to anticipate a measurable improvement in health-related quality of life. However, it may be reasonable to anticipate that the gains in convenience and access lead to gains in overall quality of life.[7]

It may be valuable to discuss several factors to keep in mind in the evaluation of telehealth programs. First, suitable outcome indicators and measures must be identified, and reliable and valid instruments to measure the socioeconomic benefit of telehealth must be developed and consistently applied. Second, relevant frameworks may need to be developed to capture monetary and nonmonetary measures in addition to any unintended consequences. Third, telehealth programs should be implemented and evaluated in a culturally aware and culturally sensitive manner. In addition, evaluations should include examination of the social, organizational, and policy aspects of telehealth.[10]

It is key to note here that consistency in measures that assess the effectiveness of a treatment modality has important implications in decision making. There are analyses where telemedicine services may be used to replace the tradition face-to-face encounters between patients and health care physicians and providers. In these cases, it may be adequate to consider disease-specific measures to estimate the effectiveness of one modality (face to face) rather than another (telemedicine). The downside to this approach is that the outcomes measures may not be generalizable if the disease-specific measures are different. With that caveat, if specific outcome measures show equal or better patient outcomes than usual care, then the next step is to assess the differences in costs using standard costing techniques.[1]

In most real-life situations, a telehealth solution is rarely a complete substitute for a face-to-face encounter; there is typically some combination of face to face and telemedicine, which requires a thorough understanding of each of the options analyzed in addition to understanding the current care pathway. Understanding the cost and benefits of an analysis is only the beginning of the decision-making process. In projecting whether a telehealth program will be a success or failure, there are additional factors that are beneficial to keep in mind: the reliability of equipment and software plus the level of technical support; political, economic, and/or budgetary issues; whether there is a perceived need for telehealth services; aptitude and ability to train the workforce and turnover levels; level of cooperation between in organizations with multiple entities or that are part of networks.[11]

VALUE OF TELEHEALTH TO THE HEALTH CARE SYSTEM

Telehealth can provide value to the health care system in a variety of ways; however, the cost-effectiveness of telemedicine may depend on many factors, including the service that is being evaluated; whether it is the physician, hospital, or patient's perspective; the type of analysis completed; how the outcomes are quantified;

how fast the technology is accepted; and the overall usage or uptake rate of the service.[1,8] In addition, the stakeholders bearing the costs may differ from those experiencing the benefits, which in most cases are patients and employers. It is important to be clear about the viewpoint chosen (provider, patient, society) for the analysis and how this affects the results.[1]

In addition to cost-effectiveness, the success of a program is also something to be considered. Success in telehealth can be taken to reflect the extent to which it makes a "sustained, worthwhile contribution to the operation of health services and the maintenance or improvement of health status."[12] The development of the information superhighway; fiber optic and broadband networks, combined with new methods to digitally compress information; and even the advent of consumer wearables and robotics with audio and visual capabilities all make it possible to provide consultations, real-time interpretation of images, and management of chronic conditions in a way that was not possible just a few years ago.[13]

Telehealth also has the ability to engage patients in their own care and this move toward engaging patients in their own care is not simply the right thing to do, it is quickly becoming the norm amid growing evidence that patient-engaged care is associated with better health outcomes, better care experience for patients, and lower health care costs. Patient-centeredness, the idea that care should be designed around patients' needs, preferences, and circumstances, is a central tenet of health care delivery. Engaged, powerful patients are central to achieving better outcomes at a better value.[5] However, telemedicine evaluations should ensure that the technology is safe and generates as much benefit as conventional means before any decision about implementation is made.[11]

Current and future physicians will need to develop competencies that will enable them to navigate this new telehealth landscape. Efforts within medical education to develop and enhance physician telehealth competency are discussed next.

VALUE OF TELEHEALTH IN MEDICAL EDUCATION

Before the COVID-19 pandemic, the American Medical Association (AMA) and other professional and regulatory bodies recognized that future physicians would need to develop competencies that would enable them to navigate a telehealth landscape. These entities encouraged medical schools across the country to accelerate the work of developing and integrating telehealth into medical school curricula. The rate of integration had remained slow but steady. According to data from the Academy of American Medical Colleges (AAMC), during the 2013 to 2014 academic year only 44% of medical schools reported having incorporated telehealth into their clerkship curricula and 27% into their preclerkship curricula (**Fig. 1**). These numbers had increased to 68% and 44% respectively as of the 2017 to 2018 academic year. The observation that medical schools had found more opportunities to include telehealth into clerkship courses is notable and likely reflects the increasing integration of telehealth into routine clinical practice. The breadth of experiences for clerkship students is also notable and ranged from unplanned exposure to telehealth during patient care to more robust exposure during structured telehealth electives. The rate of incorporation of telehealth education into preclerkship courses had lagged behind that of clerkship courses, though many schools had identified opportunities for growth. Based on 1 survey, 71% of sampled schools have incorporated didactic learning about telehealth, 53% offered real patient telehealth experiences for preclerkship students, 59% had incorporated standardized patient encounters, and 29% had incorporated telehealth exposure into student

scholarly projects.[14] Barriers to integration of telehealth in medical school curricula were numerous and reflected barriers to health care integration such as concerns regarding reimbursement, electronic medical record system capabilities and integration, privacy issues, licensure requirements, and patient satisfaction concerns.[15] At the start of 2020, it was thought that these intransigent issues would continue to create barriers for years to come, but then the COVID-19 pandemic occurred.

The COVID-19 pandemic has been a catalyst for the rapid integration of telehealth into health care delivery systems and medical education. The AAMC and individual schools of medicine are working to develop telehealth-related competency sets and reliable professional activity frameworks. Once developed, these tools will allow medical schools to define telehealth-related learning objectives and ultimately develop more robust learning activities that align with the new telehealth landscape. Some of these activities will occur in virtual patient care settings where much of primary care and subspecialty care is now occurring. For example, within the Kaiser Permanente system, more than 90% of primary care visits and greater than 50% of some subspecialty visits have been converted to virtual visits in response to the pandemic. The distinctive value-based Kaiser

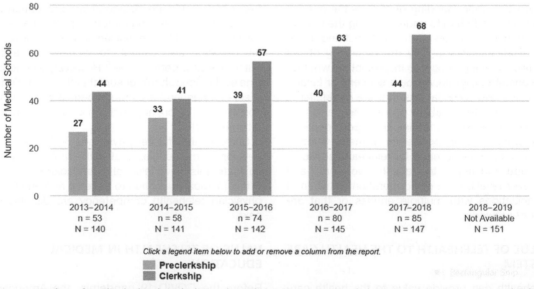

Click a legend item below to add or remove a column from the report.

■ Preclerkship
■ Clerkship

Fig. 1. Number of medical schools including telemedicine in required and elective courses. Survey item: check the topics listed that are included in the curriculum as part of a required course and/or an elective course. Note: data for telemedicine were not collected in 2018 to 2019. *n* indicates the total number of medical schools that included the topic in either a required or an elective course in the given academic year. *N* indicates the total number of medical schools that participated in the survey for the given academic year. (Source: LCME Annual Medical School Questionnaire Part II, 2013-2014 through 2018-2019. Courtesy of the American Association of Medical Colleges, Washington DC; with permission.)

Permanente model has allowed for this transition in a rapid, agile, and seamless manner. As the new Kaiser Permanente Bernard J. Tyson School of Medicine prepares to welcome its first class of students, who will begin clinical experiences within their first year, we are working to understand how we can adapt and capitalize on the virtual care transformation to deliver a unique and innovative learner experience. Other medical schools are similarly evaluating their systems to identify new telehealth learning opportunities.

Although the current pandemic has created an unprecedented opportunity to show the value of telehealth to medical education, there are important questions that need to be answered. How will medical students develop the vital clinical and emotional skills needed for future face-to-face clinical interactions? How will student development be assessed toward the telehealth competencies? Are there unforeseen equity, inclusion, and diversity-related implications for learners and patients secondary to the rapid integration of telemedicine into medical education? There are no simple answers to these questions, but the community of medical educators, led by the AAMC, have created spaces for discussion, to share best practices, and to collaborate on medical education research to address these questions.[16] Outcomes related to this collaborative work will help to determine the long-term landscape of telehealth medical education. Regardless of the exact details of that landscape, there is little doubt that medical education will be forever changed by the COVID-19 pandemic.

In response to the COVID-19 pandemic, health care organizations have accelerated their adoption of telehealth, and medical education is adapting to ensure that the next generation of physicians have the skills needed to thrive in this new telehealth environment. These trends may allow the US health care system to contain costs while continuing to provide high-quality care and more equitable health care outcomes.

REFERENCES

1. Bergmo TS. Can economic evaluation in telemedicine be trusted? A systematic review of the literature. Cost Eff Resour Alloc 2009;7(1):1–10.
2. Dávalos ME, French MT, Burdick AE, et al. Economic evaluation of telemedicine: review of the literature and research guidelines for Benefit–Cost analysis. Telemed J E Health 2009;15(10):933–48.
3. CMS historical health care expenditures. 2019. Available at: https://www.cms.gov/Research-Statistics-Data-and-Systems/Statistics-Trends-and-Reports/NationalHealthExpendData/NationalHealthAccountsHistorical. Accessed May 28, 2020.
4. Belluz J. We finally have a new U.S. maternal mortality estimate. It's still terrible. 2020. Available at: https://www.vox.com/2020/1/30/21113782/pregnancy-deaths-us-maternal-mortality-rate. Accessed May 28, 2020.
5. Cosgrove DM, Fisher M, Gabow P, et al. Ten strategies to lower costs, improve quality, and engage patients: the view from leading health system CEOs. Health Aff 2013;32(2):321–7. Available at: https://search.proquest.com/docview/1347785405.
6. McIntosh E, Cairns J. A framework for the economic evaluation of telemedicine. J Telemed Telecare 1997;3(3):132–9.
7. Snoswell C, Smith AC, Scuffham PA, et al. Economic evaluation strategies in telehealth: obtaining a more holistic valuation of telehealth interventions. J Telemed Telecare 2017;23(9):792–6.
8. Mistry H. Systematic review of studies of the cost effectiveness of telemedicine and telecare. Changes in the economic evidence over twenty years. J Telemed Telecare 2012;18:1–6.
9. Chandler D. Massachusetts institute of technology; how to predict the progress of technology. 2013. Available at: http://news.mit.edu/2013/how-to-predict-the-progress-of-technology-0306. Accessed May 30, 2020.
10. Jennett PA, Scott RE, Hall LA, et al. Policy implications associated with the socioeconomic and health system impact of telehealth: a case study from Canada. Telemed J E Health 2004;10(1):77–83.
11. Bergmo TS. Economic evaluation in telemedicine – still room for improvement. J Telemed Telecare 2010;16(5):229–31.
12. Hailey D, Crowe B. A profile of success and failure in telehealth – evidence and opinion from the successes and failures in telehealth conferences. J Telemed Telecare 2003;9(2_suppl):22–4.
13. Pelletier-Fleury N, Lanoé J, Philippe C, et al. Economic studies and 'technical' evaluation of telemedicine: the case of telemonitored polysomnography. Health Policy 1999;49(3):179–94.
14. Waseh S, Dicker A. Telemedicine training in undergraduate medical education: mixed methods review. JMIR Med Educ 2019;5(1):e12515.
15. US telemedicine industry benchmark survey. 2017. Available at: https://www.healthlawinformer.com/wp-content/uploads/2017/05/2017-telemed-us-industry-survey.pdf.
16. Resource hub, 2020 Coronavirus (COVID-19) resource hub. 2020. Available at: https://www.aamc.org/coronavirus-covid-19-resource-hub#medical education. Accessed May 13, 2020.

Printed and bound by CPI Group (UK) Ltd, Croydon, CR0 4YY

03/10/2024

01040307-0007